I0023591

A Makeover To Takeover Your Health

Research-based Smoothies

Autoimmune disorders,
Mental health wellness, and
Weight management.

Elsa-Sofia Morote, Ed.D., Ph.D.

Salud, L'Chaim, Añañau, Delish!

@copyright Elsa-Sofia Morote

All rights reserved. No part of this guide may be reproduced in any form without written permission from the publisher, except for brief quotations used in critical articles or reviews.

The photos of the smoothies and smoothie ingredients featured in this guide were captured by Elsa-Sofia Morote and are protected by copyright laws. However, you may use these photos with proper credit given to the copyright holder, Dr. Elsa-Sofia Morote. If you wish to obtain permission to use these photos or have any related inquiries, please feel free to contact Dr. Elsa-Sofia Morote

Legal & Disclaimer
The information contained in this book is not designed to replace or take the place of any form of medicine or professional medical advice. The information in this book has been provided for educational and entertainment purposes only.

The information contained in this book has been compiled from sources deemed reliable, and it is accurate to the best of the Author's knowledge; however, the Author cannot guarantee its accuracy and validity and cannot be held liable for any errors or omissions. Changes are periodically made to this book. You must consult your doctor or get professional medical advice before using any of the suggested remedies, techniques, or information in this book.

Upon using the information contained in this book, you agree to hold harmless the Author from and against any damages, costs, and expenses, including any legal fees potentially resulting from the application of any of the information provided by this guide. This disclaimer applies to any damages or injury caused by the use and application, whether directly or indirectly, of any advice or information presented, whether for breach of contract, tort, negligence, personal injury, criminal intent, or under any other cause of action.

You agree to accept all risks of using the information presented inside this book. You need to consult a professional medical practitioner in order to ensure you are both able and healthy enough to participate in this program.

ISBN: 978-0-9853714-9-4

Library of Congress Control Number: 2023920746

1st Edition

Leaf Comfy LLC, New York, USA

DEDICATION

As someone who has faced the challenges of immunological diseases, I understand the silent everyday battles of those who strive for a healthy life. This book is dedicated to those who aspire to achieve good health and aims to empower you to transform your well-being using the abundant resources of fruits, vegetables, grains, nuts, seeds, and legumes.

GET MORE FROM THIS BOOK

Unlock more valuable resources by visiting our book's official website at www.amakeovertotakeover.com. Access a treasure trove of FREE supplementary materials to enhance your reading experience and empower you on your journey. Don't miss out – explore the wealth of resources waiting for you today!

TABLE OF CONTENTS

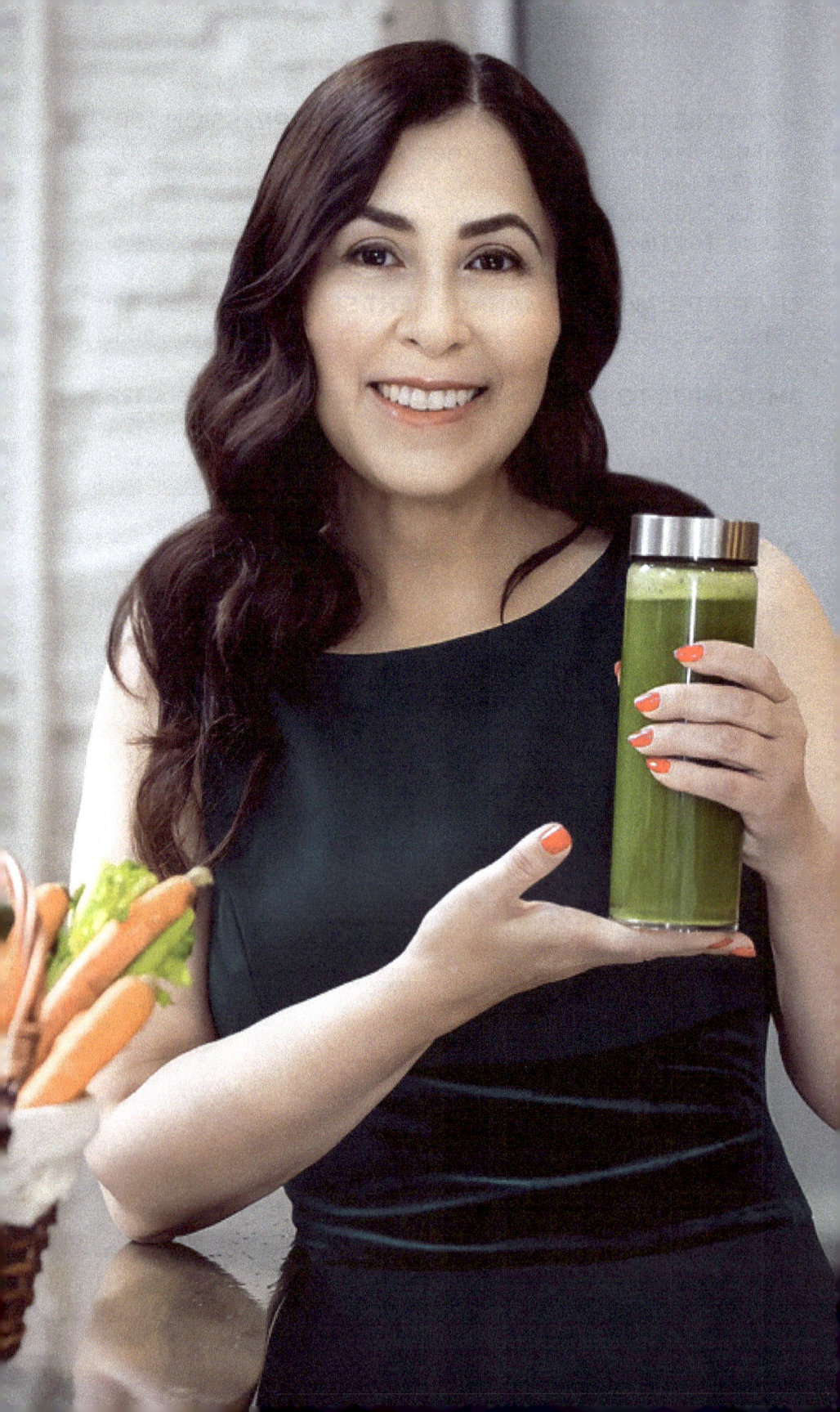

A note from
Dr. Elsa-Sofia Morote

The inspiration for this book struck me when I was conducting workshops on my previous book, "A Makeover to Takeover: Take over Your Professional Happiness". A few attendees had been with health issues and felt their quest for professional joy was being hindered by their struggle to maintain health. I sympathized with them, sharing my personal experience of managing autoimmune disorders while offering suggestions on how they could handle their health challenges. Six months later, they came back to me. They mentioned how valuable my guidance had been and pleaded with me to share my knowledge to improve others' lives.

A few months after, while hosting another talk a participant expressed concerns about weight-related discrimination during job interviews. Her doctor had recommended maintaining a healthy weight to help her better manage her diabetes. I shared healthy weight loss strategies given my personal experience of shedding 30 pounds. Half a year later, I received a grateful letter from her, accompanied by a picture. She, too, insisted that I share my insights with the world.

Prior to disseminating my knowledge to the public, I made the deliberate choice to enhance my understanding of health and nutrition. To achieve this, I enrolled in a course offered by Harvard Medical School, which was under the guidance of Dr. Beth Frates, who serves as the President of the American College of

Lifestyle Medicine.

How did I become so well-informed? Well, I suppose it all began when I was diagnosed with an autoimmune disorder, Hypothyroidism, and my desire for a normal life led me on a quest for knowledge. Living with multiple autoimmune disorders can be challenging as they often occur together and require visits to various specialists such as rheumatologists, ophthalmologists, dermatologists, and internists. These appointments are typically brief, and doctors refer patients to one another to determine the appropriate prescriptions. Medications are adjusted until an effective treatment is found, but over time, they may stop working or impact different organs, leading to the need for new medications. It becomes a cycle of ever-changing prescriptions to manage the symptoms.

While you are longing for a cure and a return to normalcy, medical doctors often inform you that autoimmune disorders have no known cure. However, you will likely come across alternative practitioners, holistic gurus, and health coaches on social media who claim to have discovered treatments. In your quest for relief, you try these various approaches, investing time and money in the process. Some treatments may provide temporary relief, while others may worsen your condition.

Having tried different approaches myself, I initially followed the prescribed medication regimen when diagnosed with my first autoimmune disorder. This condition silently affected my weight and resulted in hair loss, as well as cold hands and feet. My attempts to lose weight were complex, and doctors advised me to accept my "new normal", which I reluctantly did.

The second autoimmune disorder, Lupus, I developed was quite evident, especially on my face, prompting me to search for a remedy. I reached out to functional medicine practitioners who proposed nutrition and supplement-based approaches, and I also consulted a traditional Chinese medicine doctor who emphasized gut health and suggested dietary restrictions. While I ultimately chose not to pursue treatment with them, gaining insight into their perspectives proved valuable. I realized that with my multiple doctoral and master's degrees, I could conduct my own research.

Thus, I embarked on an extensive research endeavor, creating a spreadsheet, and databases to document my findings regarding the medications and supplements that worked best for me. Armed with this information, I approached my doctors and convinced them to prescribe the treatment I believed would be effective. Simultaneously, I made dietary changes and incorporated supplements into my routine. I kept a journal to track food, mental, and environmental triggers, and then actively avoided them. In addition to reading research-based articles, I explored non-research books and engaged in group discussions with individuals facing similar challenges. Each time I heard something new, I researched using scientific articles to validate the statements.

Chewing raw vegetables had always been a struggle for me. It wasn't until I uncovered yet another autoimmune condition (they never seem to come alone!)—Sjögren's syndrome—that I realized the cause of my reluctance to munch on leafy greens. This condition significantly reduced salivary flow, leading those with severe xerostomia to avoid crunchy foods like raw vegetables. Though raw vegetables presented a challenge for me to consume, I stumbled upon a solution: blending them into smoothies with other ingredients made them much more appealing. With determination, I summoned the courage to try my very first green smoothie, and to my utter surprise, I found it quite enjoyable. I then began implementing my self-designed treatment plan under the supervision of doctors. Remarkably, all my symptoms went into remission, and I almost forgot that I had ever been sick.

To deepen my knowledge, I enrolled in the Wellness and Nutrition course offered by Harvard Medical School. This turned out to be one of the best decisions I've ever made for myself. Each class was exceptional and reinforced the importance of making decisions based on rigorous research. It was empowering to hear the President of Lifestyle Medicine endorse this approach, and I became a passionate advocate for lifestyle medicine principles.

After completing the course and receiving certification from Harvard Medical School, I began to focus on developing my own smoothie recipes. I conducted extensive research, tested various combinations on myself, invited friends to taste and provide feedback, and carefully reviewed different additives that could enhance the nutritional value of the smoothies. I was always mindful of the price and accessibility of ingredients, ensuring that anyone could have access to them.

As I continued to refine my smoothie formulas, I noticed significant improvements in my own health, and my friends and family who tried them also experienced positive effects. I started creating customized smoothie recipes for my friends and family to address specific needs, such as cleanses, weight management, mental health, and even conditions like Parkinson's. These smoothies soon became cherished gifts for birthdays and anniversaries, and the gratitude I received through numerous thank-you notes was overwhelming.

Encouraged by the positive responses and the growing demand for my recipes, more and more people urged me to publish them.

As a researcher, professor, and higher education executive in a leadership position, I was concerned that others might perceive my health disorders as a weakness and that it could hinder my prospects for career advancement in academia. Nonetheless, my desire to help others and contribute to the well-being of humanity gradually outweighed my apprehensions. At that moment, I made the choice to share this book with the world.

Recognizing the pressing health crises surrounding immunological diseases, weight management, and mental health, I have structured this book into three chapters that address each area. My goal is to provide research-based smoothie recipes that can support individuals in achieving smoother health, just as they have helped me and many of my followers.

Strap in and prepare to enjoy these smoothies as you embark on a journey to a healthier you!

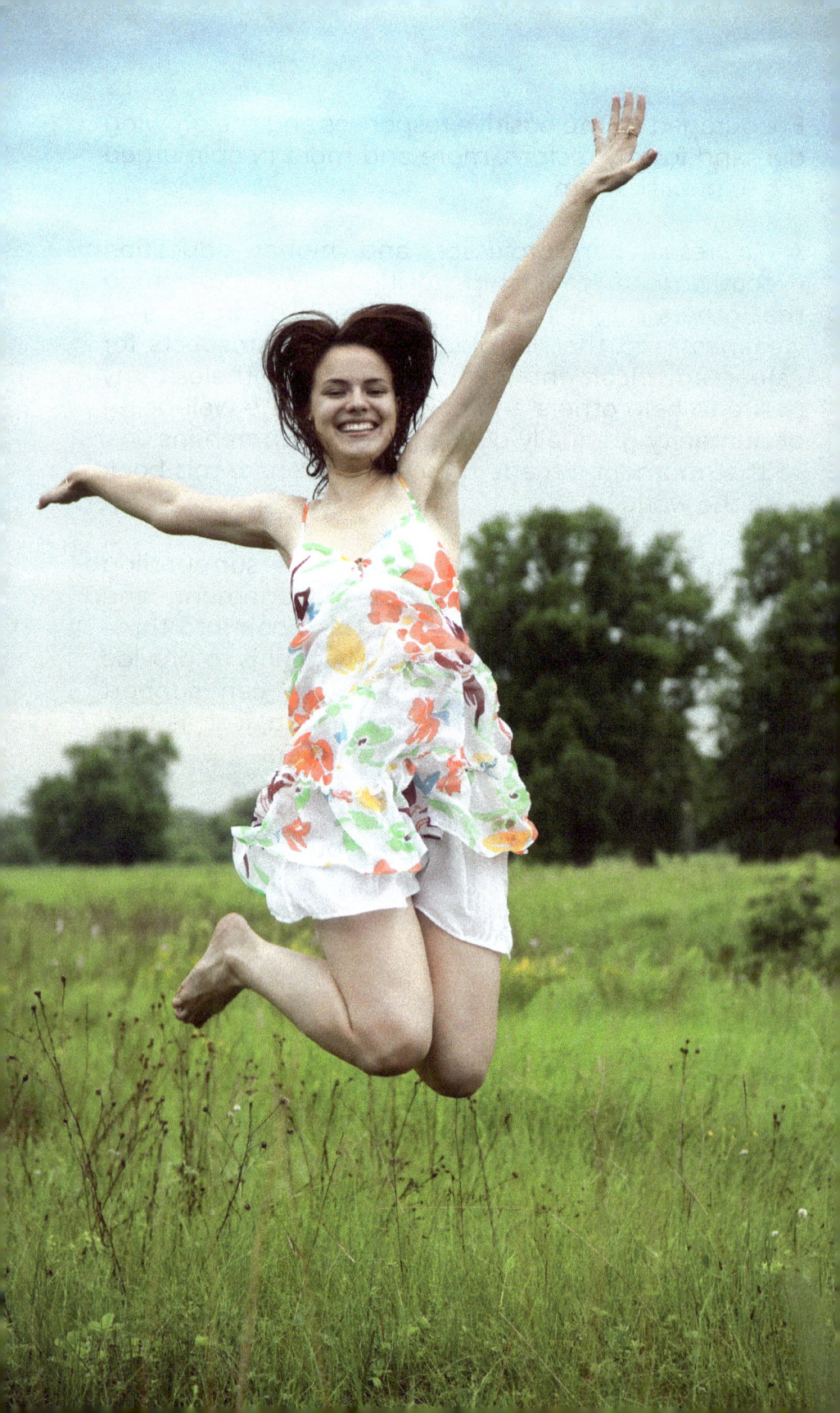

INTRODUCTION

Across the globe, there is a concerning increase in the prevalence of non-communicable diseases, including obesity, hypertension, diabetes, metabolic syndrome, chronic respiratory diseases, cancer, and more. For example, according to the Centers of Disease Control and Prevention (CDC) between 1999-2000 and March 2020, the prevalence of obesity in the United States saw a notable rise, climbing from

30.5% TO 41.9%.

Simultaneously, the occurrence of severe obesity also exhibited a significant increase, surging from

4.7% TO 9.2%

during this period. These conditions are largely influenced by the stressful and demanding lifestyle that characterizes our competitive world. Lifestyle behaviors play a significant role in the development and progression of these non-communicable diseases.

Unhealthy lifestyle choices, such as poor dietary habits, sedentary behavior, inadequate physical activity, chronic stress, and substance abuse, contribute to the development of these diseases. The consumption of processed and high-calorie foods, coupled with a lack of exercise, leads to weight gain, obesity, and metabolic disturbances. Sedentary lifestyles and a lack of physical activity further exacerbate the risk of developing chronic conditions.

Chronic stress, prevalent in today's fast-paced and competitive environment, also plays a detrimental role in the onset of non-communicable diseases. Prolonged exposure to stress hormones can disrupt various physiological processes, including blood pressure regulation, immune function, and metabolic balance, thus contributing to hypertension, cardiovascular diseases, and other related conditions.

Moreover, the use of tobacco, excessive alcohol consumption, and exposure to environmental toxins can significantly increase the risk of developing certain cancers, respiratory diseases, and other chronic illnesses.

Research has provided us with a number of evidence-based methods and strategies for promoting a healthy lifestyle. These approaches include maintaining regular physical activity, adopting a balanced and nutritious diet, ensuring sufficient sleep, managing stress, fostering social connections, and avoiding risky substances. Lifestyle medicine emphasizes the use of scientific evidence to prevent, treat, and reverse chronic diseases. This rise in non-communicable diseases highlights the urgent need for individuals to adopt healthier lifestyle behaviors. Thankfully, science has provided us with a number of evidence-based methods and strategies for promoting a healthy lifestyle. These approaches include maintaining regular physical activity, adopting a balanced and nutritious diet, ensuring sufficient sleep, managing stress, fostering social connections, and avoiding risky substances. Lifestyle medicine emphasizes the use of scientific evidence to prevent, treat, and reverse chronic diseases.

Public health initiatives and policies aimed at promoting healthy lifestyles and creating supportive environments can also contribute to reducing the burden of non-communicable diseases.

The COVID-19 pandemic highlighted the importance of virtues such as solidarity and moral responsibility. It also underscored the significance of positive relationships characterized by kindness, compassion, and empathy. These virtues guide individuals in making choices that prioritize their genuine needs over mere desires. For example, individuals aiming to stay physically active and prevent obesity need to exercise self-control to avoid unhealthy eating habits [1].

By practicing self-care, temperance, and solidarity with others, individuals can avoid vices such as illicit drugs, excessive alcohol consumption, unhealthy food choices, or smoking, which contribute to cardiovascular or respiratory diseases. Similarly, companies that prioritize justice, safety, and social responsibility create an environment that supports healthy choices and well-being for their employees and stakeholders [1].

The 6 Pillars of Lifestyle Medicine

Nutrition
Evidence supports the use of a whole food, plant-predominant diet to prevent, treat and reverse chronic illness.

Physical Activity
Regular, consistent physical activity is an important part of overall health and resiliency.

Stress Management
Managing negative stress can lessen anxiety, depression and immune dysfunction and leads to improved well-being.

Sleep
Improving sleep quality can improve attention span, mood, insulin resistance and can reduce hunger, sluggishness and more.

Social Connection
Positive social connections have beneficial effects on physical, mental, and emotional health.

Avoid Risky Substances
The use of tobacco and excessive alcohol consumption have been shown to increase the risk of chronic diseases and death.

The six pillars of lifestyle medicine encompass various aspects of well-being. Plant-based nutrition, following guidelines such as the Mediterranean-Dietary, Approach to Systolic Hypertension (DASH), and Intervention for Neurodegenerative Delay (MIND), can reduce the risk of chronic diseases like Alzheimer's disease. Regular physical activity not only promotes physical health but also helps prevent neurocognitive decline. Managing stress, improving sleep quality, and fostering social connections have positive effects on mental, emotional, and cognitive well-being. Additionally, avoiding risky substances like tobacco and excessive alcohol consumption reduces the risk of chronic diseases and premature death [2].

Engaging in regular physical activity may also help in preventing neurocognitive decline. The evidence for prioritizing physical activity and exercise researched and universally recommended as first-line therapy for many chronic diseases as well as for prevention [3]. Moreover, physical exercise can boost energy expenditure and enhance endurance [2] [3].

Conversely, high levels of perceived stress in adulthood and the use of substances such as alcohol, nicotine, and opioids have been linked to an increased risk of mild cognitive impairment and dementia. Furthermore, poor sleep quality and social isolation have been associated with a more rapid decline in cognitive function [1]

These findings highlight the significant impact of lifestyle changes on an individual's health. Therefore, prioritizing these lifestyle factors can empower individuals to take proactive steps in safeguarding their health. My personal advice is to strongly consider the six pillars of lifestyle medicine [2] to have a successful health life.

ABOUT MAKEOVER TO TAKEOVER SERIES

A book published early called "A Makeover to Takeover" outlines a six-step process towards achieving professional happiness: Perceive, Prepare, Present, Position, Promote and Persuade. Now, I aim to apply these six steps to help you optimize your health. I have now structured a three-pronged strategy for health and wellbeing: Nourish your Mind, Nourish your Body, and Nourish your Soul. This methodology has been designed to help you take control of your wellness journey.

"A Makeover to Takeover your Health: Research-based Smoothies" is divided into three 'N's (Nourish your Mind, Nourish your Body, and Nourish your Soul). The first 'N', Nourish your Mind, encapsulates the first two Ps of the makeover process: Perceive and Prepare. This involves boosting your self-awareness and outlining a blueprint for success. You will learn how to identify your strengths, areas for improvement, and how to craft an excellent wellness plan.

The second 'N' is Nourish your Body. In this stage, you will implement your wellness plan by focusing on nutrition, exercise, and restful sleep. The final 'N', Nourish your Soul, concerns maintaining your emotional health and cultivating positive social connections.

Nourish your Mind.

Perceive yourself. To optimize your health, you need to be your most significant advocate. To achieve this, it's vital to gain an understanding of your physical and mental health. Regular physical examinations can help as you'll be able to maintain a record of your health status. Not only that, an updated health history also helps your doctor track any changes or developments in your health. Physical examinations involve various tests and checks to ensure your overall health.

Prepare yourself. Design a plan to achieve your health goals. Whether you use a planner or pen and paper, the essential part is to document your goals.

Nourish your Body.

Present yourself as the healthy individual you aspire to be. Understanding the needs and strengths of your body will guide you on how to best nourish it. Make informed decisions about what to consume and avoid (such as harmful substances like drugs, alcohol, or other toxins).

Position yourself as a healthy individual who makes conscious choices. Carefully plan your nutrition, exercise, and sleep routines.

Nourish your Soul.

Promote yourself. You are now prepared to promote the new and healthier you – you are taking over your health. Learn to allocate quality time for yourself, manage stress, and practice meditation.

Persuade. Surround yourself with individuals who will support your new healthy lifestyle. It's also important that you maintain consistency in your efforts. Remember, you've got this!

"A Makeover to Takeover your Health: Research-based Smoothies" is far from your average smoothie recipe compilation. It comprises a collection of carefully curated recipes, founded on extensive research and a keen eye for premium ingredients. Detailed insights into my research can be found under the "health benefits" section.   I've made a concerted effort to make things simple for you by providing measurements and portions that are typically enough for one to two servings.

The book is segmented into three pivotal chapters:

» **Chapter 1:** Targeting Autoimmune Disorders - Lupus, Sjogren's, Parkinson's & Hashimoto's

» **Chapter 2:** Mental Health Wellness - Focusing on Depression, Anxiety & Brain Fog

» **Chapter 3:** Weight Management Strategies - Cleanse, Weight Loss & Diabetes Management.

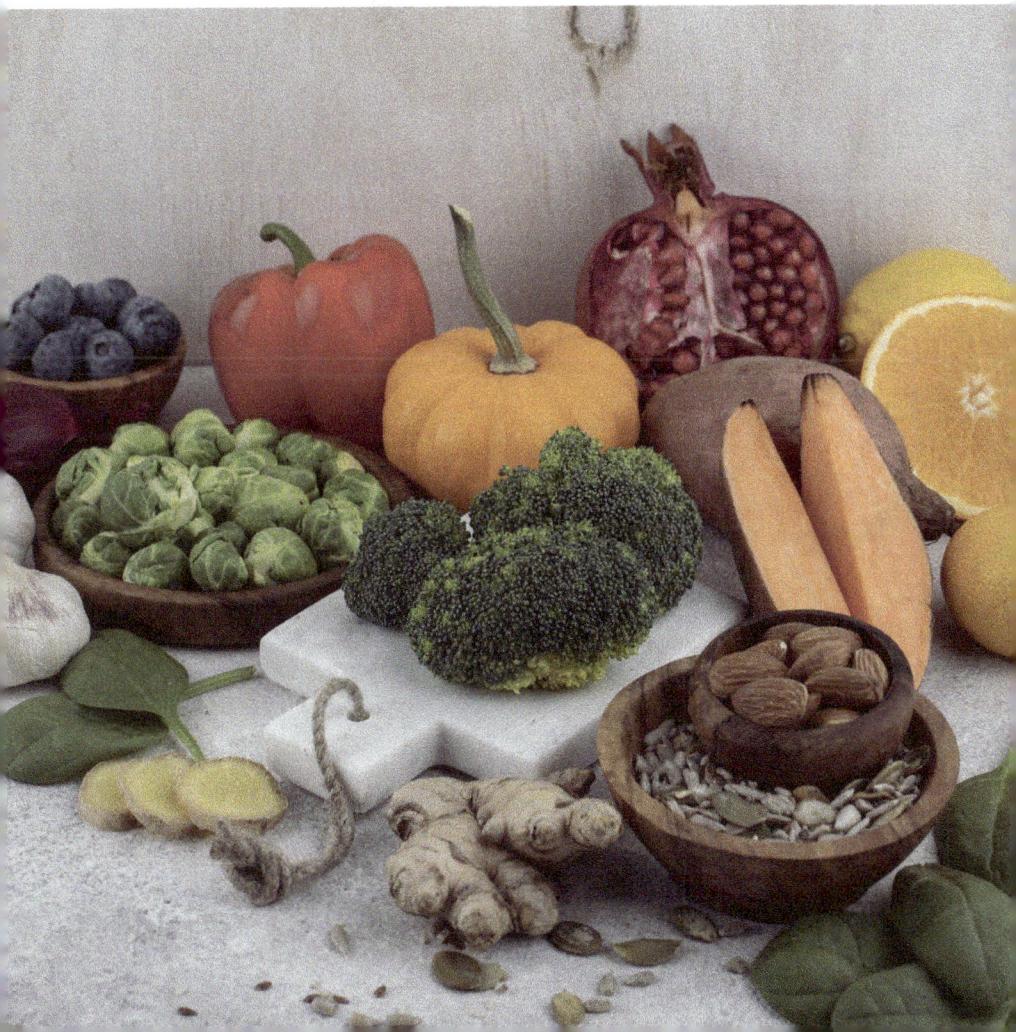

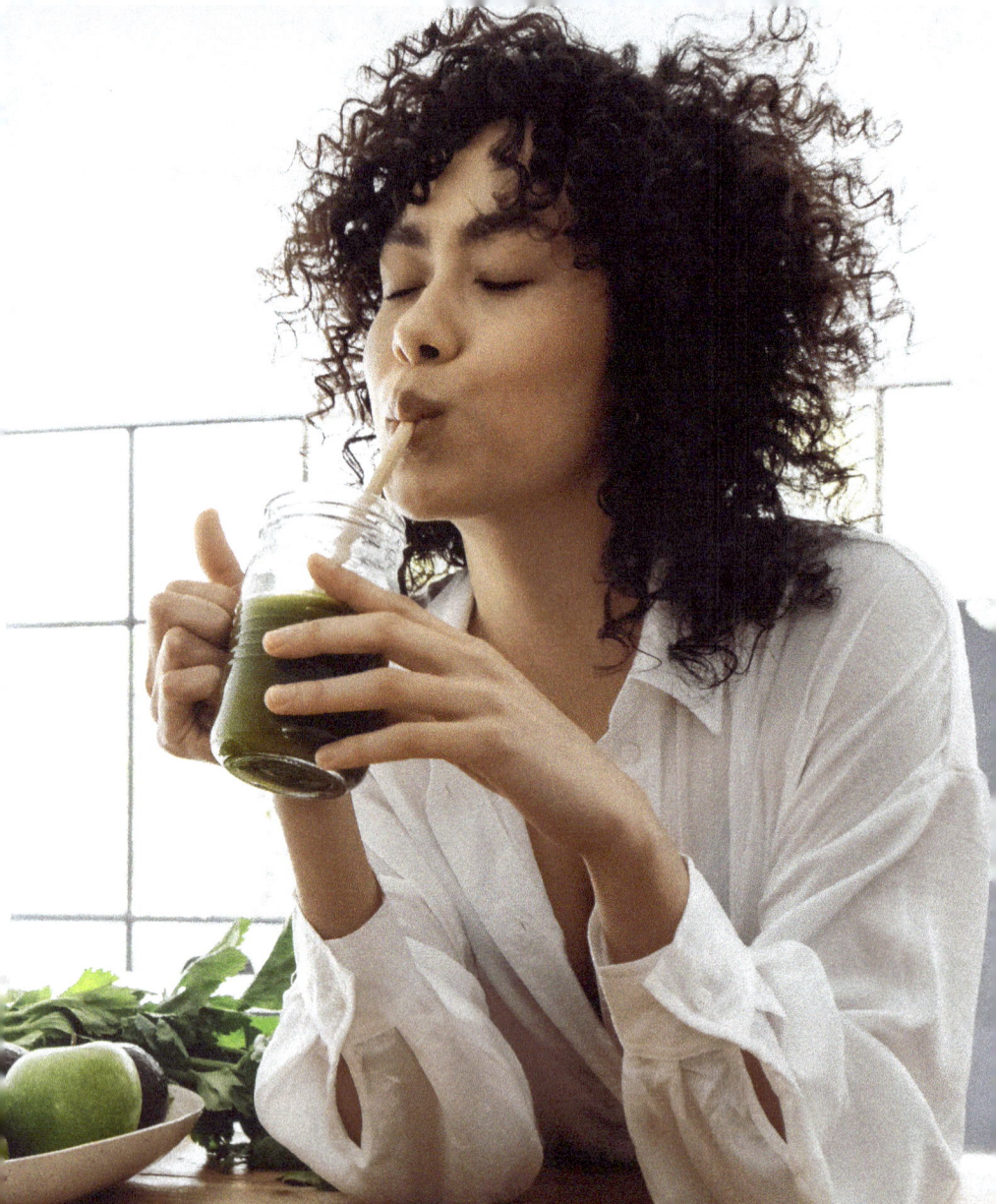

CHAPTER 1

SMOOTH AUTOIMMUNE DISORDERS

Inflammation plays a critical role in the onset of chronic illnesses. The assortment of macronutrients and the proportion of omega-6 to omega-3 fatty acids in a person's diet can have a significant impact on the activation of inflammation-associated genes [4]. Embracing an anti-inflammatory diet is essential in fighting off silent inflammation, and this includes adding omega-3 fatty acids and polyphenols, like those present in Maqui, into your daily food intake. One of the key goals of an anti-inflammatory diet is to keep insulin levels in check while reducing the intake of omega-6 fatty acids.

This chapter includes six smoothies (three anti-inflammatories and three immune boosters) and two juices. You'll need a blender for the smoothies and a juice extractor for the two juices.

Below you can find a description of the smoothies and juices that are designed to support your fight with autoimmune disorders.

AI: Anti-inflammatories

AI1. **Chocolate Purple Magic.** This smoothie presents a delightful blend of powerful anti-inflammatories and antioxidants. The enchanting purple hue is courtesy of the antioxidant-rich blueberries, while the inflammation-reducing almonds work their magic. Cocoa not only adds a luscious flavor but also aids in lowering blood pressure, and maca contributes to improved mood.

AI2. **Amber Love De-Puffiness.** Brimming with goodness from pineapple, this is a treasure trove of vitamins and minerals. Macadamia nuts join the mix to combat inflammation, while papayas enhance antioxidant absorption. Mango supports cell growth, and golden berries contribute their anti-inflammatory prowess. Ginger adds a zing with its potent anti-inflammatory and antioxidant properties.

AI3. **Pink Anti-Inflammatory Smoothie.** The incredible duo of curcumin-rich turmeric and black pepper unite to fight inflammation. Berries add a burst of antioxidants, while manuka honey showcases diverse bioactivities, including anti-inflammatory and anti-diabetic effects. Meanwhile, the green leaves, spinach, and collard greens, provide a nutrient-packed punch with their high antioxidant content.

AI4. **Green Anti-Inflammatory Smoothie.** Packed with enthusiasm, this vibrant blend stars the dynamic combination of ginger, pineapple, turmeric, and honey, teaming up to combat inflammation like champions! Collard greens and spinach join the party, thus fueling your metabolism and showering you with potent antioxidants, ready to take on cancer. Plus, the superhero manuka honey supports white blood cells in eliminating harmful toxins. Sip your way to revitalized health!

IB: Immune Boosters

IB1. **Tropic C Booster.** A tropical paradise loaded with vitamin C-rich fruits like kiwi, mango, and pineapple. Ginger and lemon join the mix to provide extra antioxidants, and chia seeds add a healthy boost. To further customize, blend with your favorite green leaf, such as spinach or Kale (note: steam the kale if you have autoimmune diseases).

IB2. **Eternal Youth Green Smoothie.** Featuring collard greens known for their diabetes-fighting properties. Almond milk, banana, and apple come together, and a touch of date provides probiotics and antifungal benefits. Moringa also offers anti-aging benefits.

IB3. **Purple Sweet Potato Regulation.** This smoothie is backed by research for its immune-modulating effects. Combined with maca and healing manuka honey, this concoction packs a powerful punch. Banana adds antioxidant, anti-diabetic, and anti-inflammatory benefits to make it a true powerhouse.

IB4. **Explore the world of healing juices with my juice extractor creations:**

- IB41. Try the invigorating **"Lady in Red"** juice, featuring beetroots, carrots, celery, and green apples with a touch of turmeric and ginger. A dash of black pepper and cinnamon adds extra antioxidants. Vegetable juices offer probiotics, and celery aids in combating obesity.

- IB42. Unleash the **"Purple Man"** vegetable juice, an antioxidant-rich blend of carrots, purple cabbage, and cucumber, promoting a healthy gut microbiota. Ginger and curcumin team up to combat inflammation, while lemon adds antimicrobial benefits. Apples provide polyphenols that act as powerful antioxidants, protecting against environmental damage.

With these delightful and healthful smoothies and juices, you can nourish your body with a burst of natural goodness and embrace a wellness journey like never before.

SHOPPING LIST TO SMOOTH AUTOIMMUNE DISORDERS

Berries: Blueberries, blackberries, strawberries, acerola cherries, maqui berries (Some of these berries you can find it frozen or in powder)

Fruits: Banana, pineapple, mango, kiwi, green apple, avocado

Greens: Spinach, collard greens or kale (steam the kale if you have a thyroid related disease), English cucumber, purple cabbage

Roots: Ginger, turmeric, beetroot, carrot

Additives: Maca powder, cinnamon, cacao powder (or dark chocolate bar), flax seeds grounded, chia seeds

Liquid: Almond milk, coconut milk, water, ice cubes

Nuts: Almond, macadamia, or hazelnut

Others: Cinnamon, black pepper, lemon juice

Sweeteners: Raw honey or organic agave or organic vanilla extract or manuka honey

ANTI-INFLAMMATORY SMOOTHIES

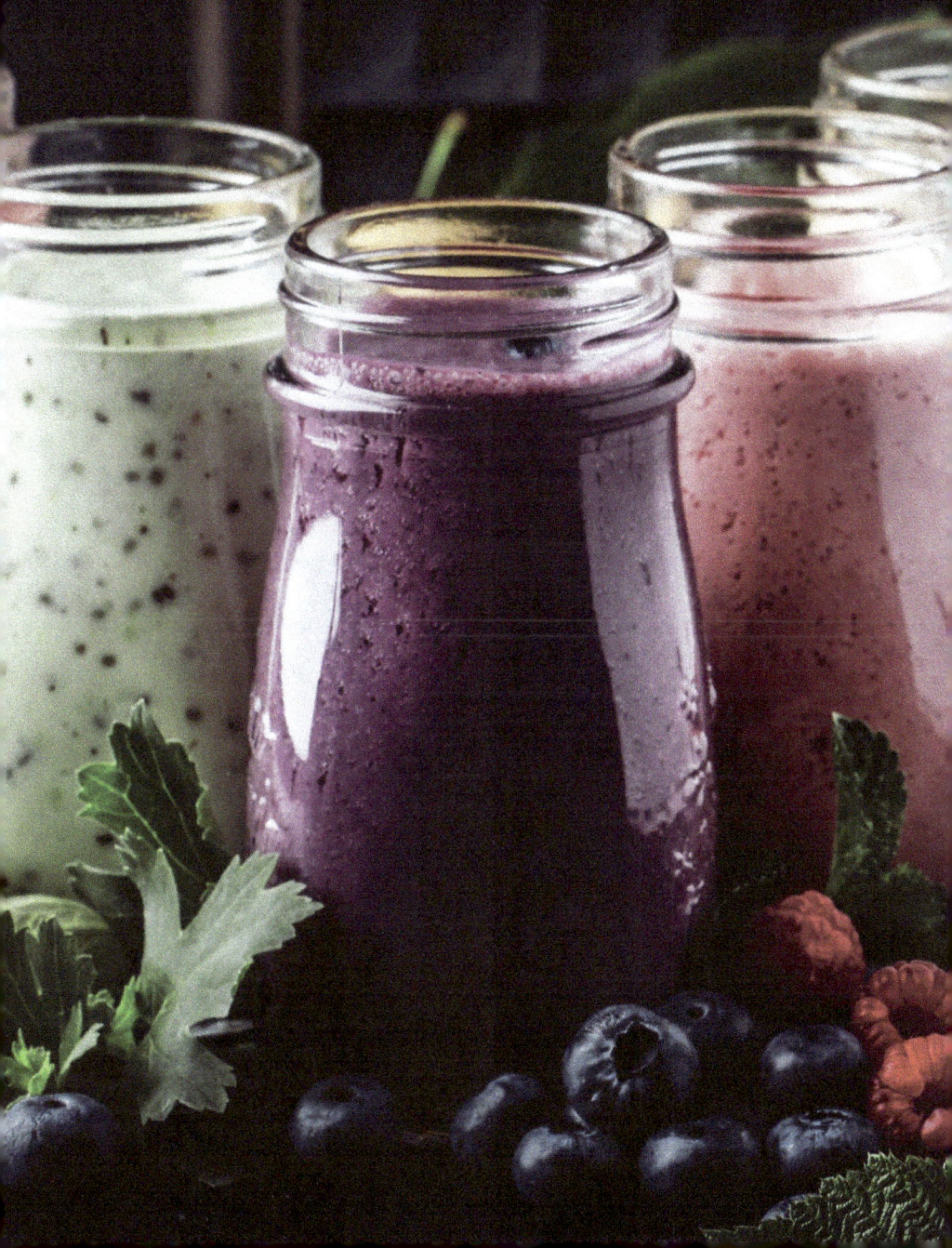

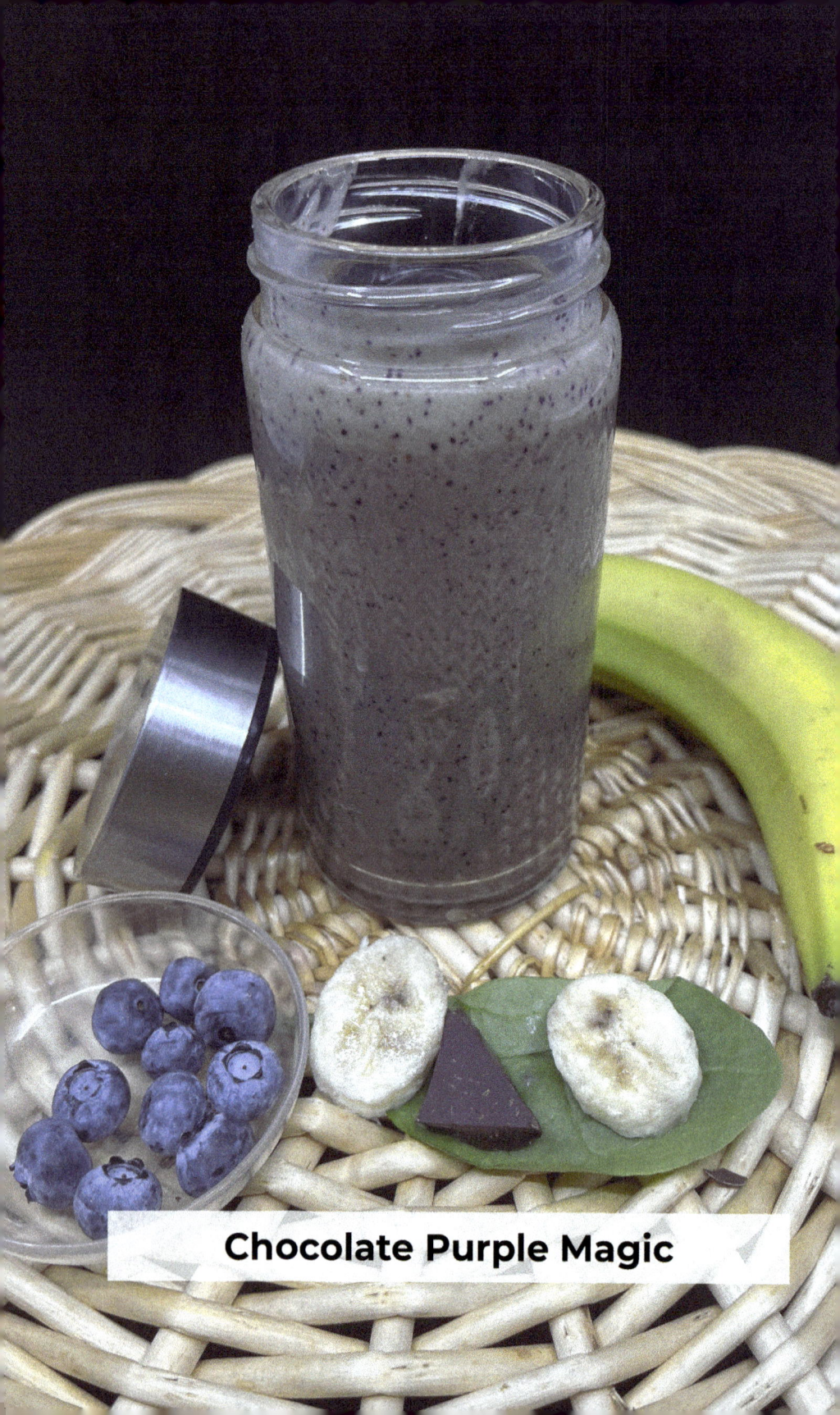

Chocolate Purple Magic

AI1. Chocolate Purple Magic

A delightful fusion of potent anti-inflammatories and antioxidants form the basis of this enchanting purple smoothie. The rich hue is a gift from antioxidant-rich blueberries, while the inflammation-reducing almonds work their magic. To add to its allure, cocoa not only imparts a luscious flavor but also aids in lowering blood pressure, while maca contributes to uplifting mood and well-being.

INGREDIENTS

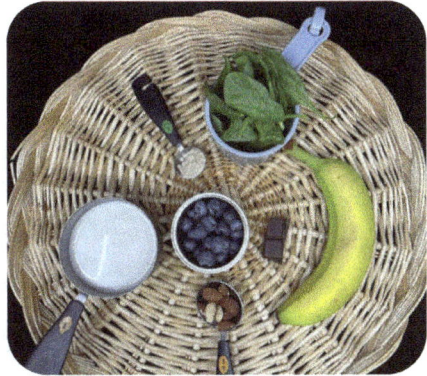

(Serves 1)

» ½ cup blueberries
» 1/2 banana
» 1 cup fresh spinach
» 7-10 almonds
» 1 teaspoon maca powder
» 1 pinch cinnamon
» 2 tablespoons cacao powder or 1 square of a dark chocolate bar
» 1 cup of water or almond milk
» 1/3 cup of ice or 5 ice cubes

INSTRUCTIONS

1. Add all of the ingredients in a blender and then blend them until smooth.
2. Then use 1 cup of water or almond milk to change the consistency as per your taste.

Chocolate Purple Magic's Ingredients

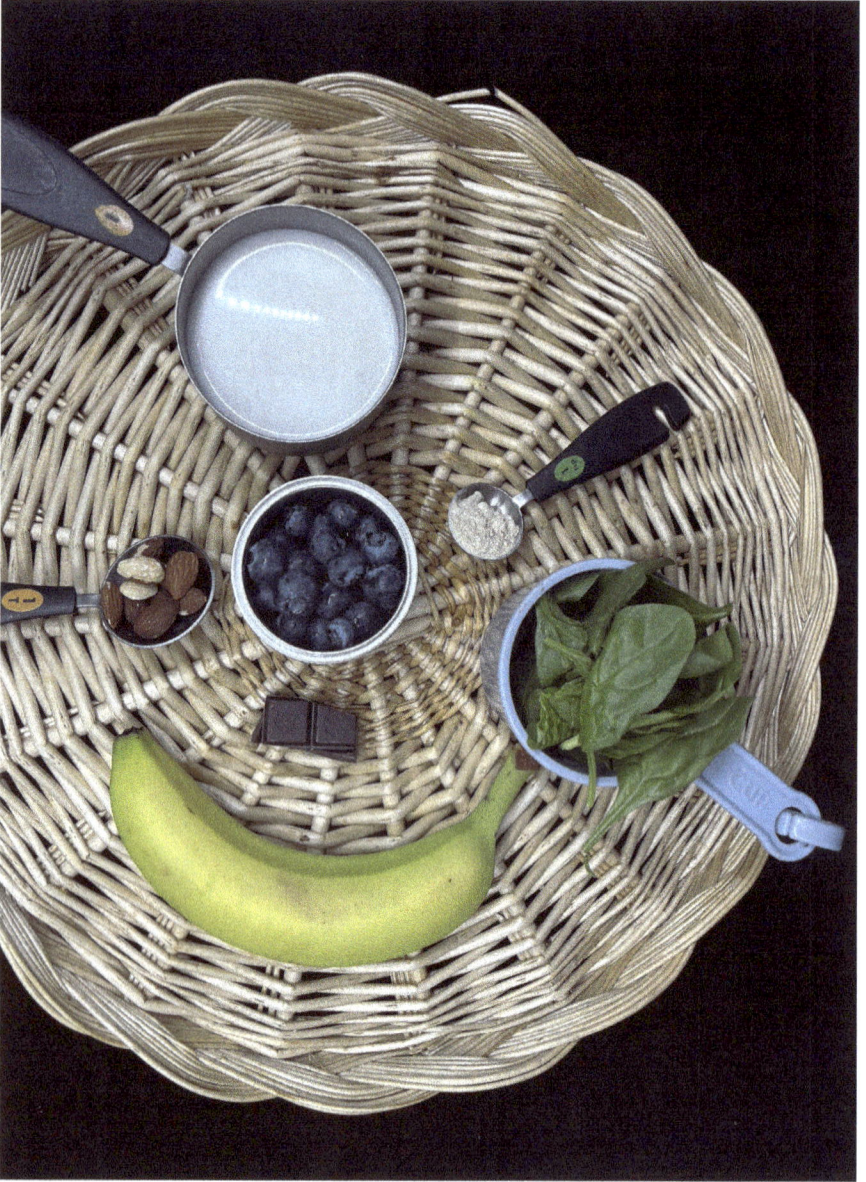

Chocolate Purple Magic nutrition facts and health benefits

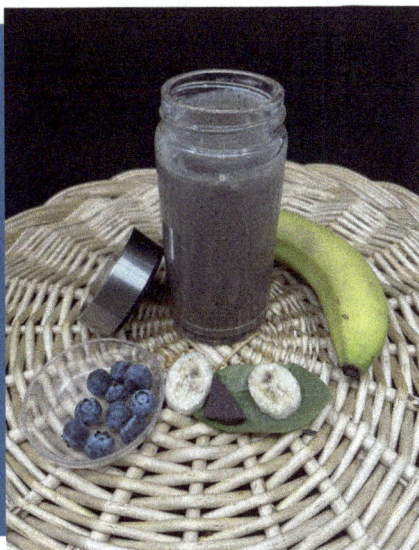

**NUTRITION FACTS
(1 serving)**

Calories: 319kcal
Carbohydrates: 58g
Protein: 8g
Fat: 9g
Saturated Fat: 0.6g
Cholesterol: 0mg
Sodium: 131mg
Potassium: 1041mg
Fiber: 12g
Sugar: 10g

HEALTH BENEFITS: Blueberries are believed to have one of the highest antioxidant levels of all common fruits and vegetables. Anthocyanins play the most important role in health benefits of blueberries. A 2022 analysis of 16 clinical trials including over 800 participants found that eating up to 60g (about 2.25 oz.) of almonds per day reduced two different markers of inflammation in the body [5]. Zeaxanthin and lutein in spinach work to prevent macular degeneration and cataracts, which are major causes of blindness [6]. Phytol, a diterpene alcohol found in chlorophylls, has been shown to potentially enhance lipid and glucose metabolism, suggesting it could have beneficial effects on health, However if you have Refsum disease you should avoid using spinach, and try different greens instead [7]. Many health advantages from cocoa have been reported, including lowered blood pressure, decreased cholesterol and blood sugar levels, enhanced blood flow, and reduced inflammation [8]. According to a 2015 study, treatment with 3.3 grammes of maca per day for six weeks improved depressive symptoms compared to a placebo treatment in 29 postmenopausal Chinese women [9].

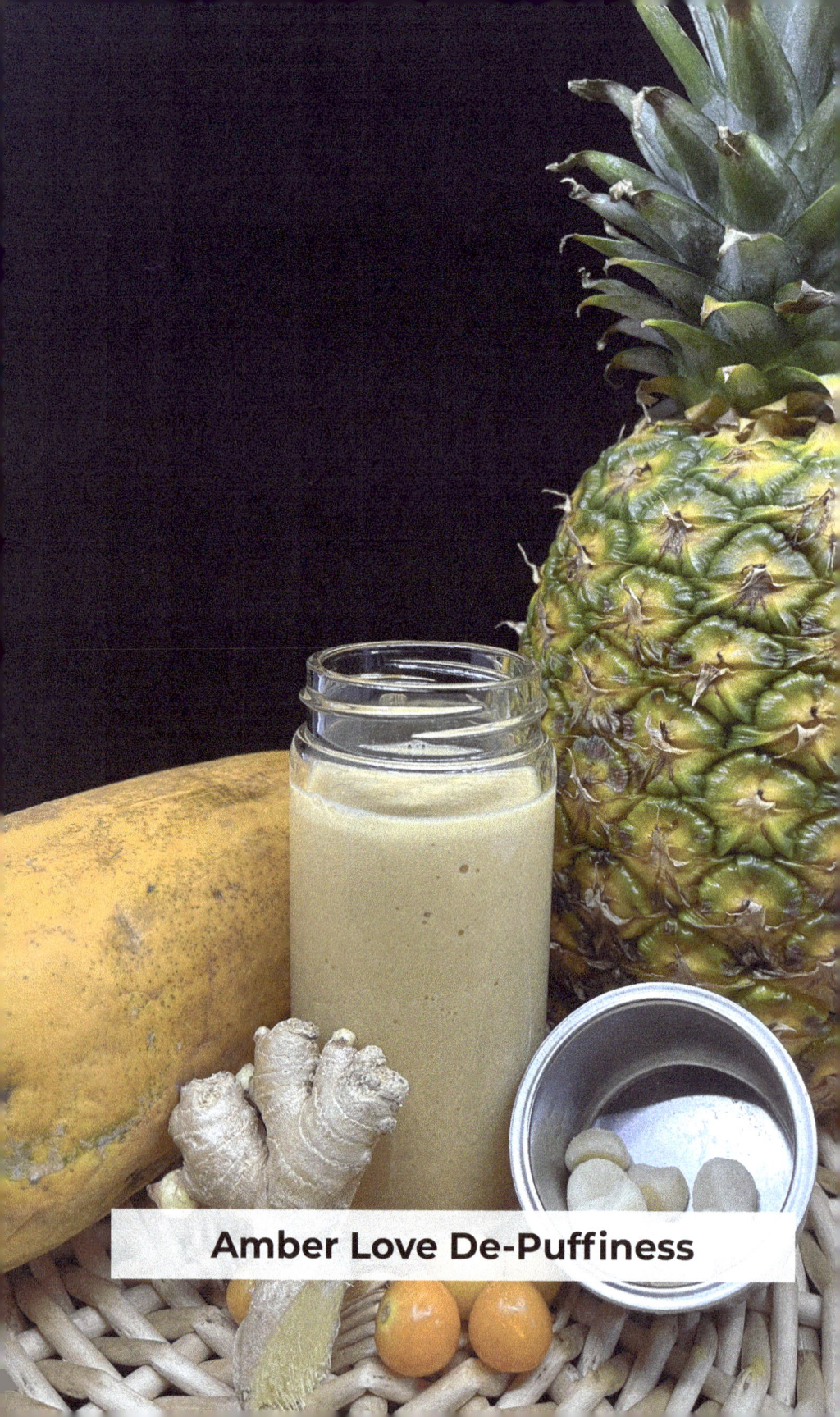

Amber Love De-Puffiness

AI2. Amber Love De-Puffiness

Overflowing with goodness, this vibrant blend showcases the treasure trove of vitamins and minerals found in pineapple. Complementing this bounty, macadamia nuts join forces to combat inflammation, while papayas step in to enhance antioxidant absorption. Meanwhile, mango plays a pivotal role in supporting cell growth, and the inclusion of golden berries brings their anti-inflammatory prowess to the mix. Adding a zing to this medley, ginger also contributes its potent anti-inflammatory and antioxidant properties, making this smoothie a true powerhouse of health benefits.

INGREDIENTS

(Serves 2)

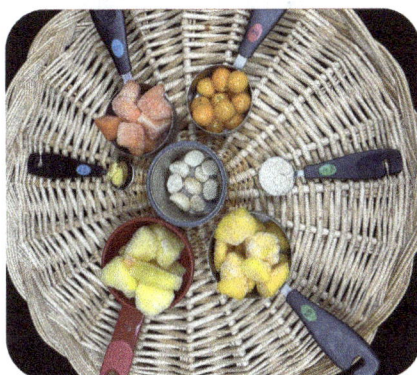

» ½ cup pineapple chucks
» ½ cup mango chunks or 1 mango
» 1/2 cup papaya chunks
» 7-10 macadamia nuts or hazelnuts
» 1/4 cup acerola cherries or golden cherries
» 1/3 teaspoon of ginger chunks
» 1 teaspoon of maca
» 1 date for sweetness (or 1 spoon of honey) (optional)
» 1 ½ cup of water
» 1/3 cup of ice or 5 ice cubes

INSTRUCTIONS

1. Place all of the ingredients into your blender and then blend smoothly.
2. Use water or almond milk to change the consistency as per your taste.
3. BON APPETITE!

Amber Love De-Puffiness's Ingredients

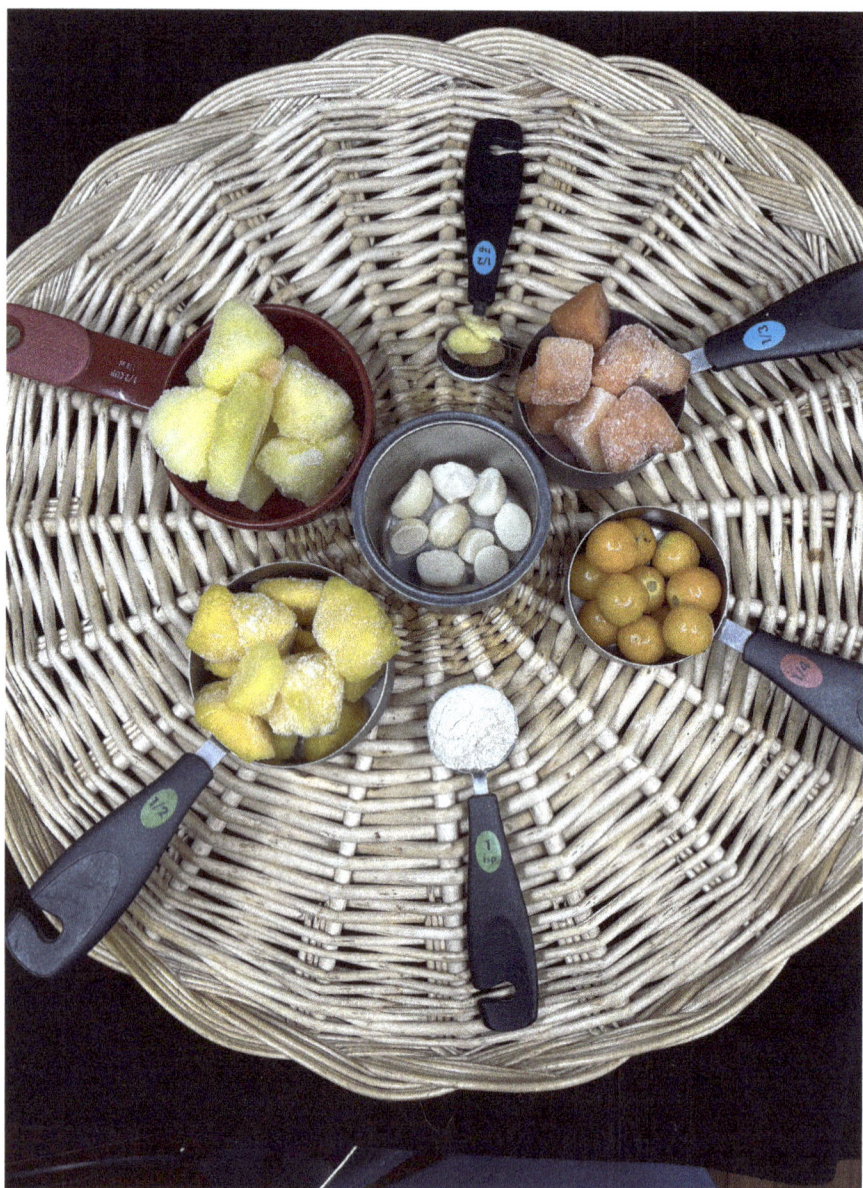

Amber Love De-Puffiness nutrition facts and health benefits

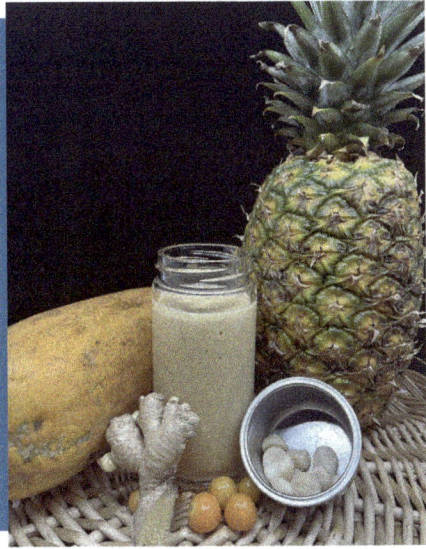

NUTRITION FACTS
(1 serving)

Calories: 462kcal
Carbohydrates: 19g
Protein: 6.4g
Fat: 23g
Saturated Fat: 3.7g
Cholesterol: 0mg
Sodium: 12.4mg
Potassium: 901mg
Fiber: 10g
Sugar: 56g

HEALTH BENEFITS: Pineapples contain other micronutrients, such as copper, thiamine, and vitamin B6, which are essential for healthy metabolism [10]. Macadamia nuts boast some of the highest flavonoid levels of all tree nuts. This antioxidant fights inflammation and helps lower cholesterol [11]. What's more, your body better absorbs these beneficial antioxidants from papayas than other fruits and vegetable [12]. Just one cup (165 grammes) of fresh mangoes provides about 67% of the daily value (DV) for vitamin C, which is one of its most astounding nutritional benefits. This water-soluble vitamin supports cell growth and repair, as well as aids in iron absorption, and strengthens your immune system [13]. Acerola surpassed all others in a study of various fruits containing vitamin C and their relative levels, especially when grown organically. According to reports, the fruit even has more vitamin C than oranges and strawberries [14]. Consumption of golden berries (Physalis peruviana L.) might reduce biomarkers of oxidative stress [15].

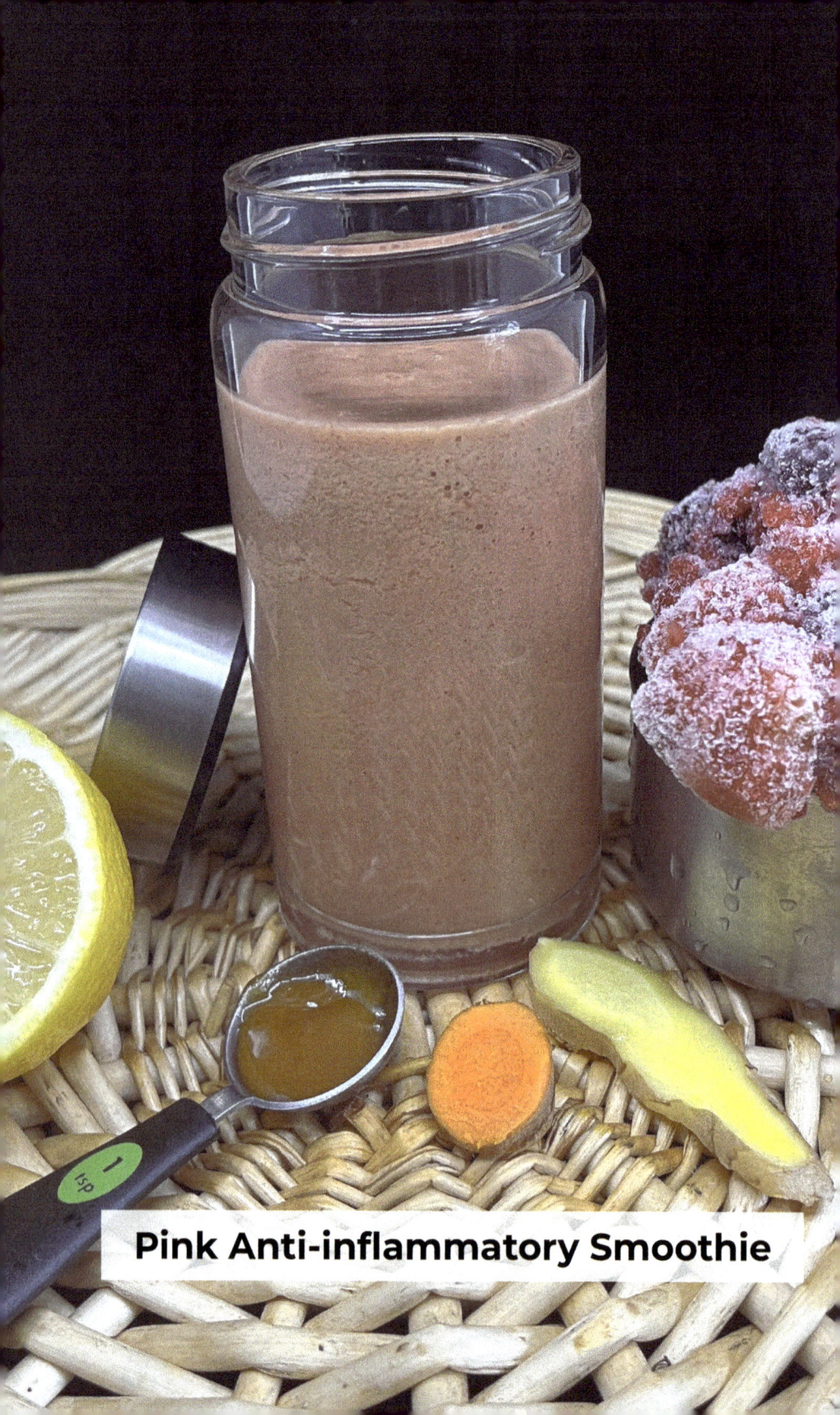
Pink Anti-inflammatory Smoothie

AI3. Pink Anti-inflammatory Smoothie

In this delicious smoothie, turmeric's curcumin and black pepper unite to fight inflammation. Berries bring antioxidants, while manuka honey offers diverse bioactivities, including anti-inflammatory and anti-diabetic effects. Spinach and collard greens deliver a nutrient-packed punch with high antioxidant content. It really is a powerful blend for overall health.

INGREDIENTS

🍽 **(Serves 2)**

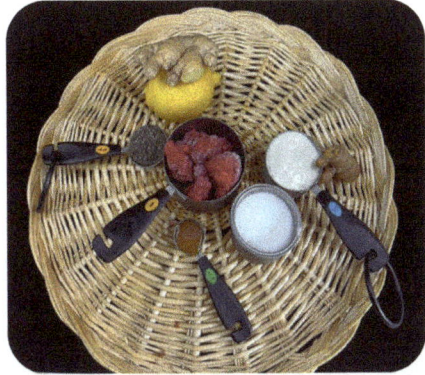

» 2 cups mixed berries frozen (or swap them for any single berry of choice)
» 1 lemon squeezed (replace it with lime juice if you prefer)
» 1 teaspoon high-quality raw honey or manuka honey if you're not on a keto diet
» 1 tablespoon chia seeds or flaxseeds
» 2 tablespoons ginger root or 4 slides of ginger root
» 1-2 tablespoons turmeric root or 3 slides of turmeric root
» 1 pinch of black pepper
» ½ cup yogurt alternative
» ¼ cup unsweetened coconut milk (optional) if not add water
» 1/3 cup of ice cubes or 5 ice cubes

INSTRUCTIONS

1. Blend all the ingredients in a blender until smooth and creamy. Do NOT strain!
2. Then, pour it into two glasses filled with ice cubes and enjoy.

Pink Anti-inflammatory Smoothie's Ingredients

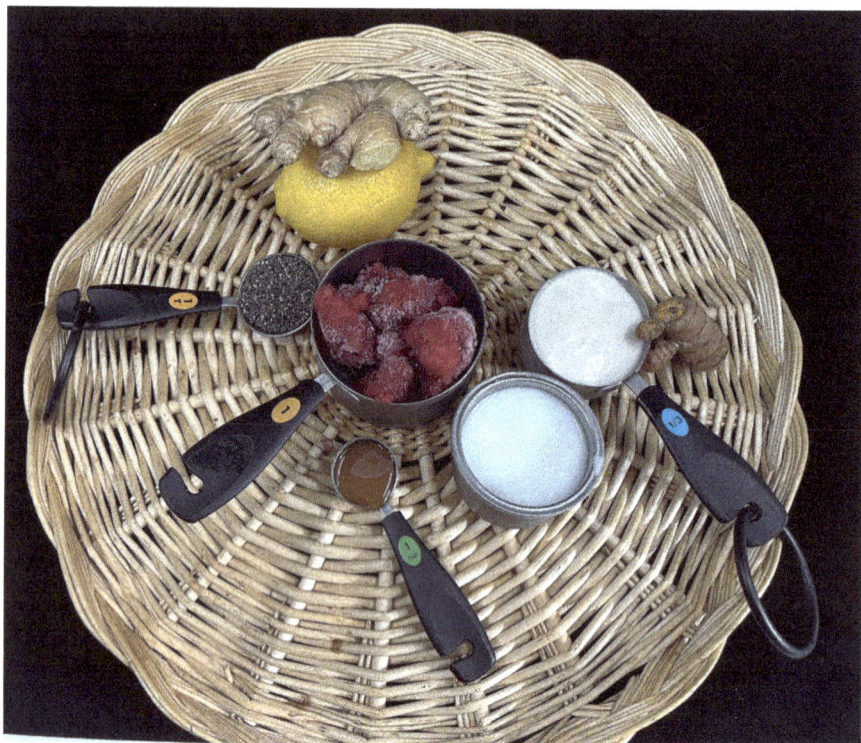

Pink Anti-inflammatory Smoothie nutrition facts and health benefits

NUTRITION FACTS
(per serving)

Calories: 188kcal
Carbohydrates: 19.6g
Protein: 9.5g
Fat: 9.3g
Saturated Fat: 3.2g
Cholesterol: 17.5mg
Sodium: 24.9mg
Potassium: 313.2mg
Fiber: 4.9g
Sugar: 9.9g

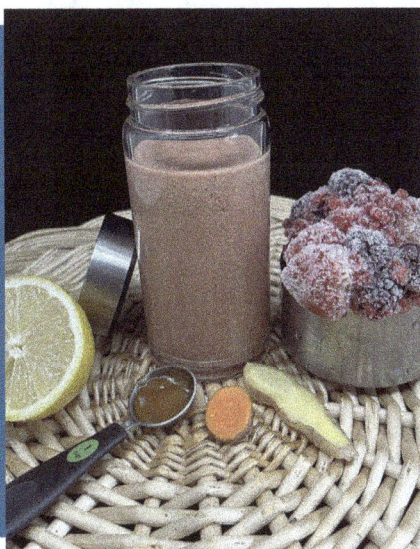

HEALTH BENEFITS: Berries are a great source of antioxidants, such as anthocyanins, ellagic acid, and resveratrol. In addition to protecting your cells, these plant compounds may reduce the risk of disease [16]. Curcumin is a popular bioactive substance for fighting inflammation [17]. Black pepper's piperine improves curcumin absorption, thus making it easier for your body to utilize it [18]. The nutrients in chia seeds may promote heart health, support strong bones, and improve blood sugar management [19]. Gingerol, a compound with potent anti-inflammatory and antioxidant effects, is abundant in ginger [20]. Honey has diverse bioactivities, including antioxidant, antimicrobial, antidiabetic, anti-inflammatory, and anticancer properties, have also made it an aspirant natural product for therapeutic applications [21]. When comparing the total antibacterial, antibiofilm, and anti-virulence activities of all the tested honeys, manuka honey demonstrated the greatest levels of these properties [22].

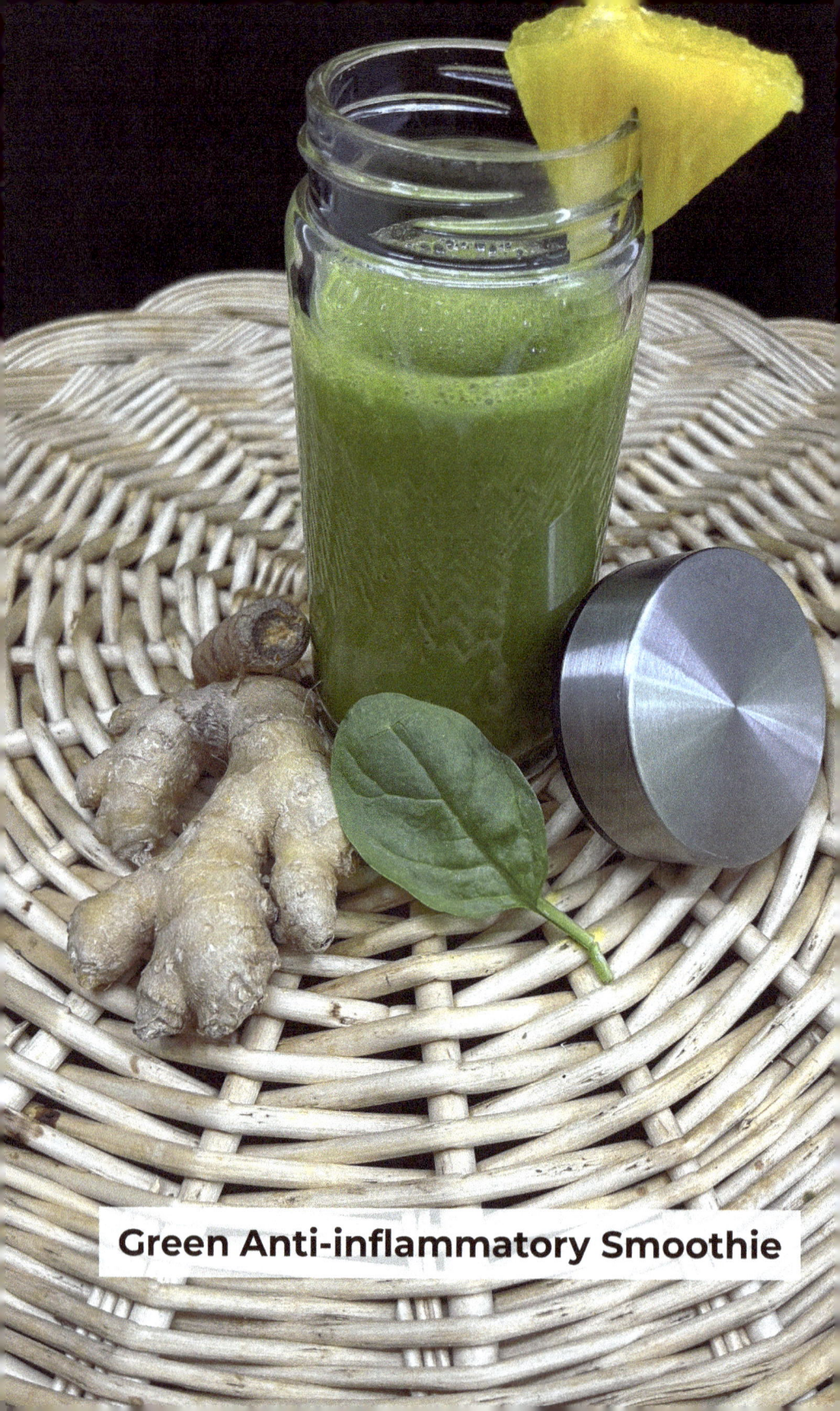
Green Anti-inflammatory Smoothie

AI4. Green Anti-inflammatory Smoothie

Experience the vibrant Green Anti-Inflammatory Smoothie, an exhilarating fusion of ginger, pineapple, turmeric, and honey to battle inflammation. Collard greens and spinach deliver nourishing nutrients, fostering a healthy metabolism while empowering your body with cancer-fighting. The journey to renewed vitality and wellness never tasted so good!

INGREDIENTS

(Serves 2)

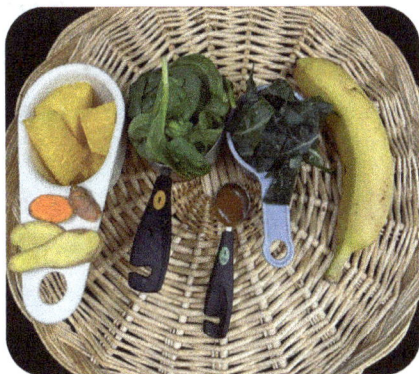

» 1 cup frozen (or not) ripe banana
» 1 cup frozen (or not) pineapple
» 1 cup organic spinach
» 1 cup collard greens
» 2 slices of ginger root
» 2 slices of fresh turmeric root
» 1 teaspoon of manuka honey or raw honey
» 1/8 teaspoon freshly ground black pepper (or just a couple of grinds)
» 1/2 cup almond milk (if you don't have almond milk then use filtered water)
» 1 cup of water and 1/3 cup of ice cubes or 5 ice cubes.

INSTRUCTIONS

1. In a large high-powered blender, add all of the ingredients along with 1 cup of water.
2. Then blend on high for 1-2 minutes or until all ingredients are well combined.
3. If necessary, add in more almond milk to thin the smoothie. BON APPETITE!

Green Anti-inflammatory Smoothie's Ingredients

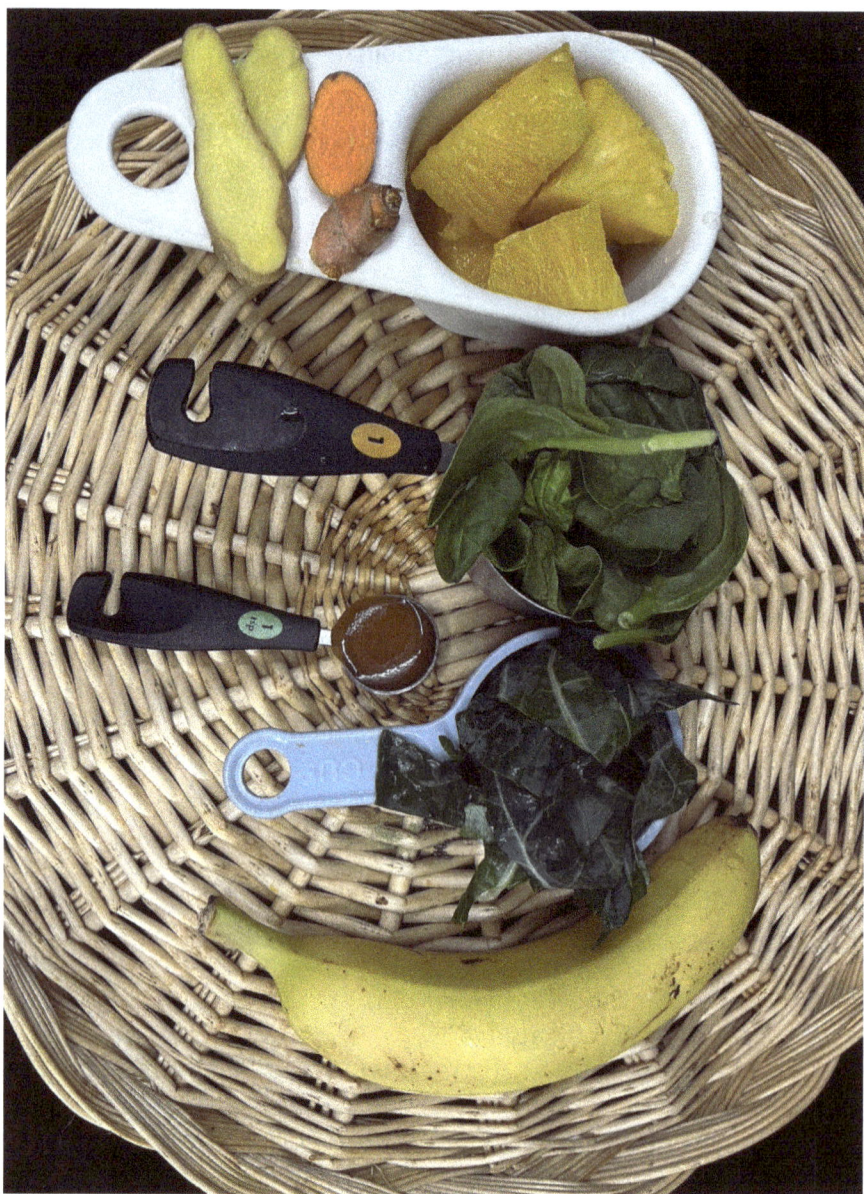

Green Anti-inflammatory Smoothie nutrition facts and benefits

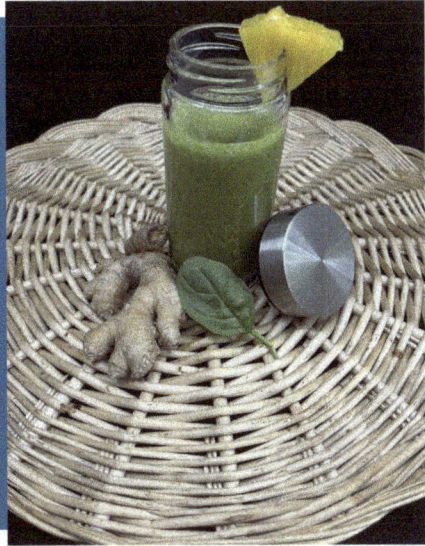

NUTRITION FACTS
(1 serving)

Calories: 253kcal
Carbohydrates: 61g
Protein: 4.4g
Fat: 3g
Saturated Fat: 0.2 g
Fiber: 7.6g
Sugar: 38.6g

HEALTH BENEFITS: Pineapple contains a number of micronutrients, such as copper, thiamine, and vitamin B6, which are essential for a healthy metabolism [10]. Spinach packs high amounts of antioxidants, which may also help to fight cancer [23]. Moreover, zeaxanthin and lutein in spinach work to prevent macular degeneration and cataracts, which are major causes of blindness [24]. Ginger is packed with gingerols, paradols, sesquiterpenes, shogaols, and zingerone, all of which have powerful anti-inflammatory and antioxidant properties [6]. Curcumin is a well-known bioactive substance that can fight inflammation [25]. In 2020, a study exploring how manuka honey can strengthen the immune system produced optimistic findings. According to the study, manuka honey enhanced the release of cytokines, which are essential for maintaining a healthy immune system. These cytokines aid white blood cells in locating and eliminating contaminated or damaged tissues [26].

IMMUNE BOOSTER SMOOTHIES

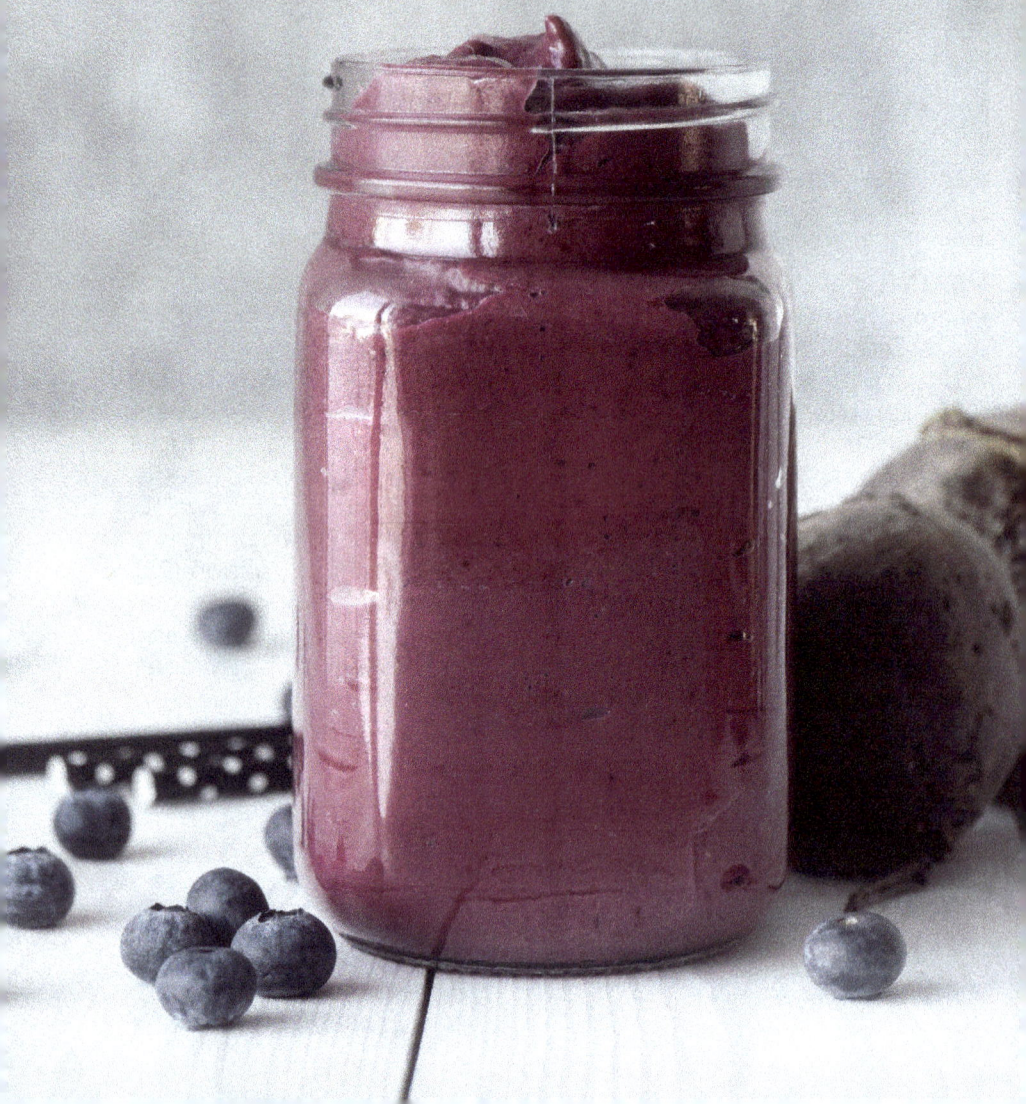

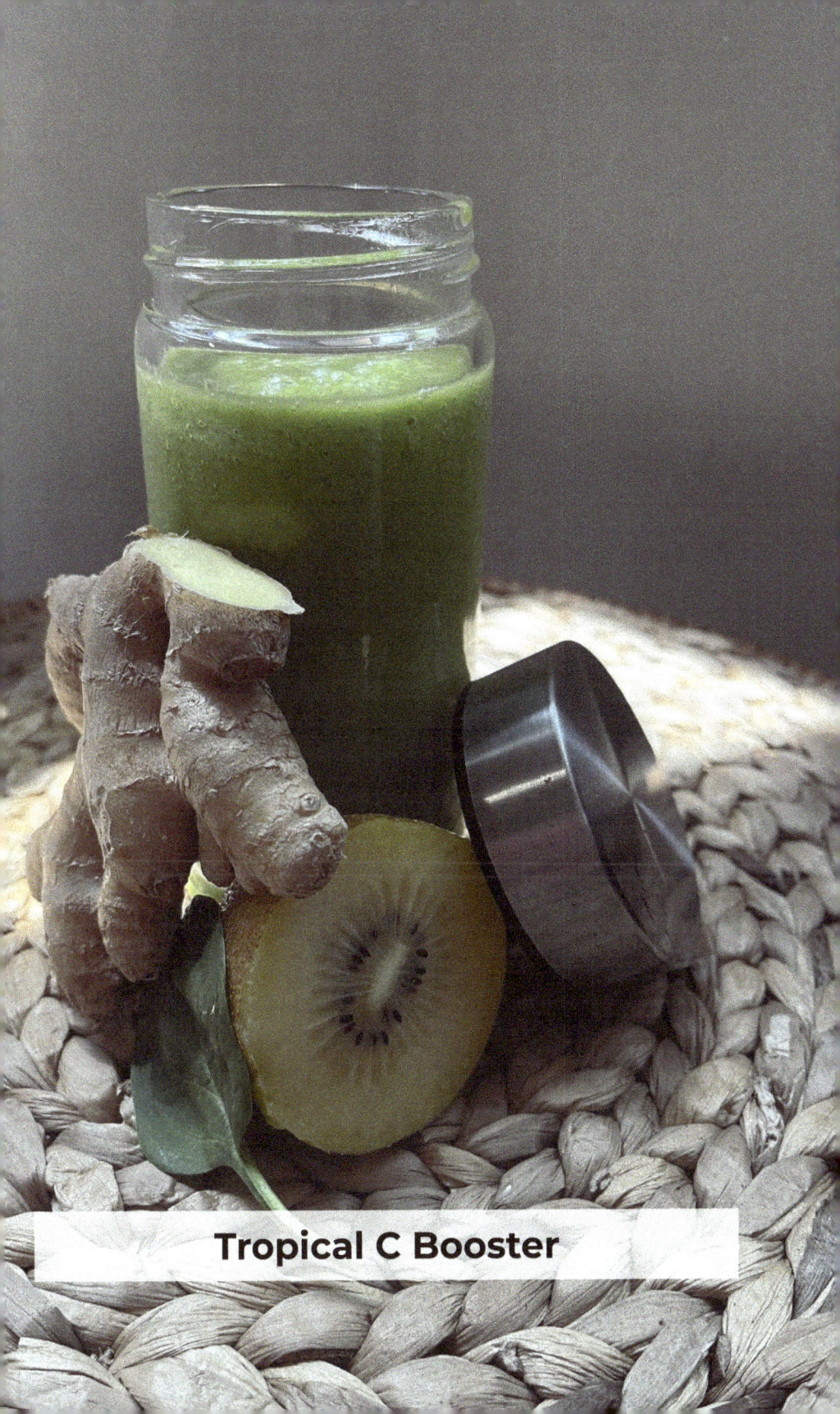
Tropical C Booster

IB1. Tropical C Booster

Indulge in a tropical paradise of Vitamin C-rich kiwi, mango, and pineapple. Infused with ginger and lemon for extra antioxidants and enhanced with chia seeds for a healthy boost. Personalize it with your favorite green leaf like spinach (or steam kale for autoimmune conditions). A truly refreshing, customizable delight awaits!

INGREDIENTS

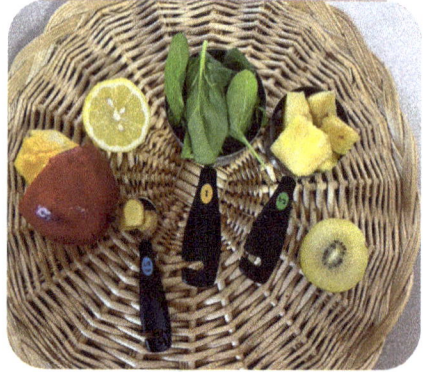

🍽 (Serves 1)

- » 1 cup roughly chopped spinach and kale (steamed), packed tightly
- » 1 ½ cups frozen mix of mango, pineapple, and kiwi chunks (or ½ mango, ½ kiwi, ¼ cup pineapple)
- » ½ teaspoon freshly grated ginger or two slides of fresh ginger
- » ½ lemon, juiced
- » ½ tablespoon chia
- » 1 ½ cups unsweetened almond milk
- » Optional: 1 date

INSTRUCTIONS

1. Add the spinach and kale to a blender with the Almond milk and blend well.
2. Then add the frozen fruit, ginger and lemon and blend until smooth. If the smoothie is too thick, add some more almond milk 1 tablespoon at a time until it's thin enough.
3. If using fresh fruit instead of frozen, reduce the almond milk amount to 1 cup and slowly add more to make your preferred thickness. Or, add 5 ice cubes before blending.
4. BON APPETITE!

Tropical C Booster's Ingredients

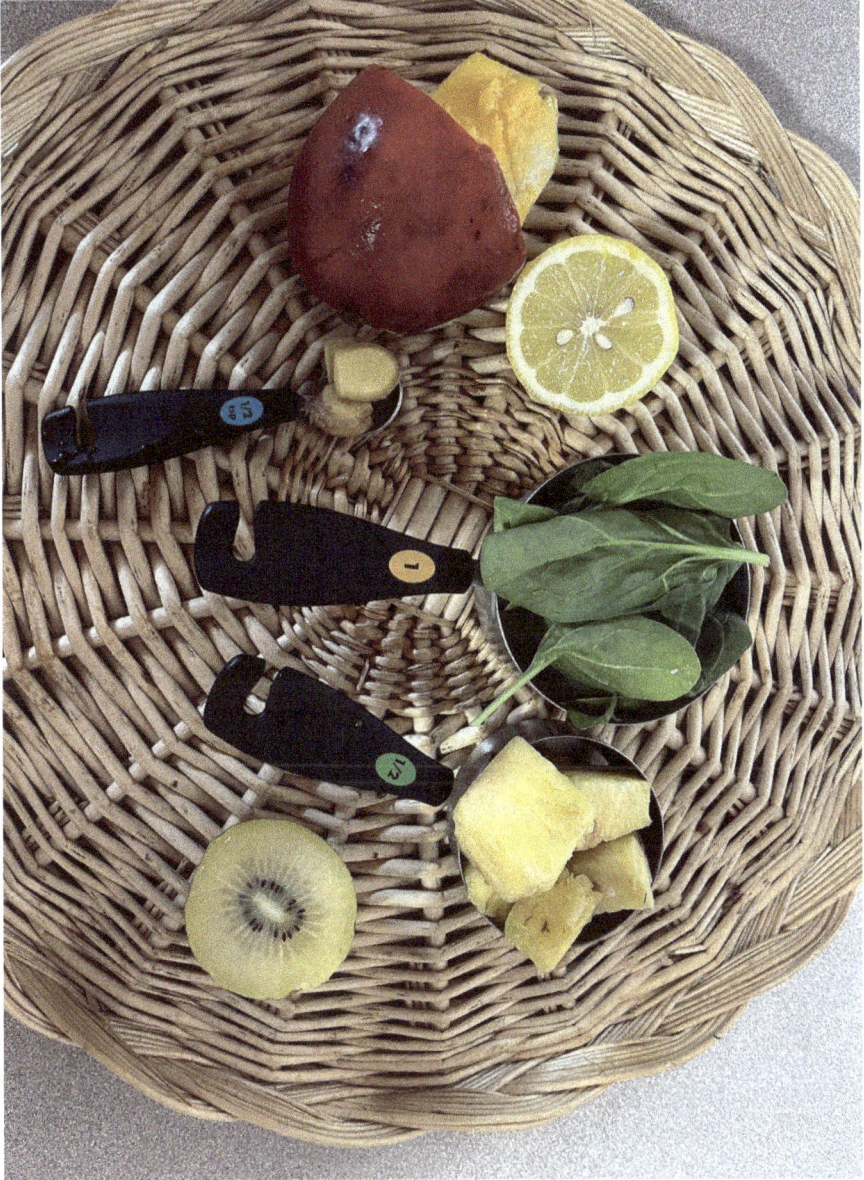

Tropical C booster nutrition facts and health benefits

NUTRITION FACTS
(1 serving)

Calories: 112kcal
Carbohydrates: 22g
Protein: 3g
Fat: 3g
Saturated Fat: 1g
Cholesterol: 0mg
Sodium: 257mg
Potassium: 329mg
Fiber: 4g
Sugar: 18g

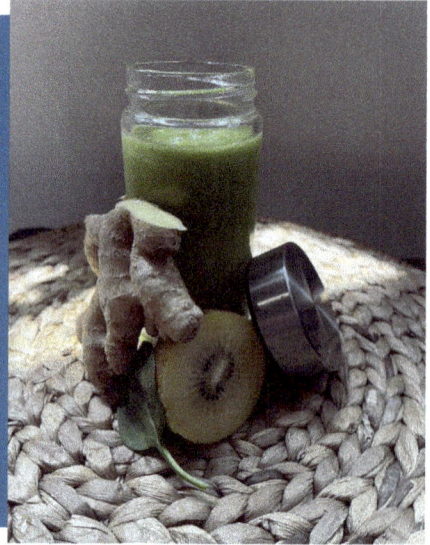

HEALTH BENEFITS: Spinach packs high amounts of antioxidants, which may also fight cancer [23]. Zeaxanthin and lutein in spinach work to prevent macular degeneration and cataracts, which are major causes of blindness [24]. Ginger is packed with gingerols, paradols, sesquiterpenes, shogaols, and zingerone, all of which have powerful anti-inflammatory and antioxidant properties [6]. Almond milk might be a good choice if you're worried about acne and want to clear up your skin. This is due to the fact that several types of almond milk are superior providers of vitamin E. Strong antioxidant vitamin E may aid in the body's removal of potentially harmful free radicals that could harm your skin [8]. Kiwi contains a peptide called kissper which is highly effective in preventing intestinal inflammation [27]. BMI scores, waist circumference, and body weight were significantly lower in male mango consumers when compared with non-consumers [28]. Eating pineapple during an infection could help to interfere with the pathogen attaching and thus help prevent the virus from getting into the host cell [29].

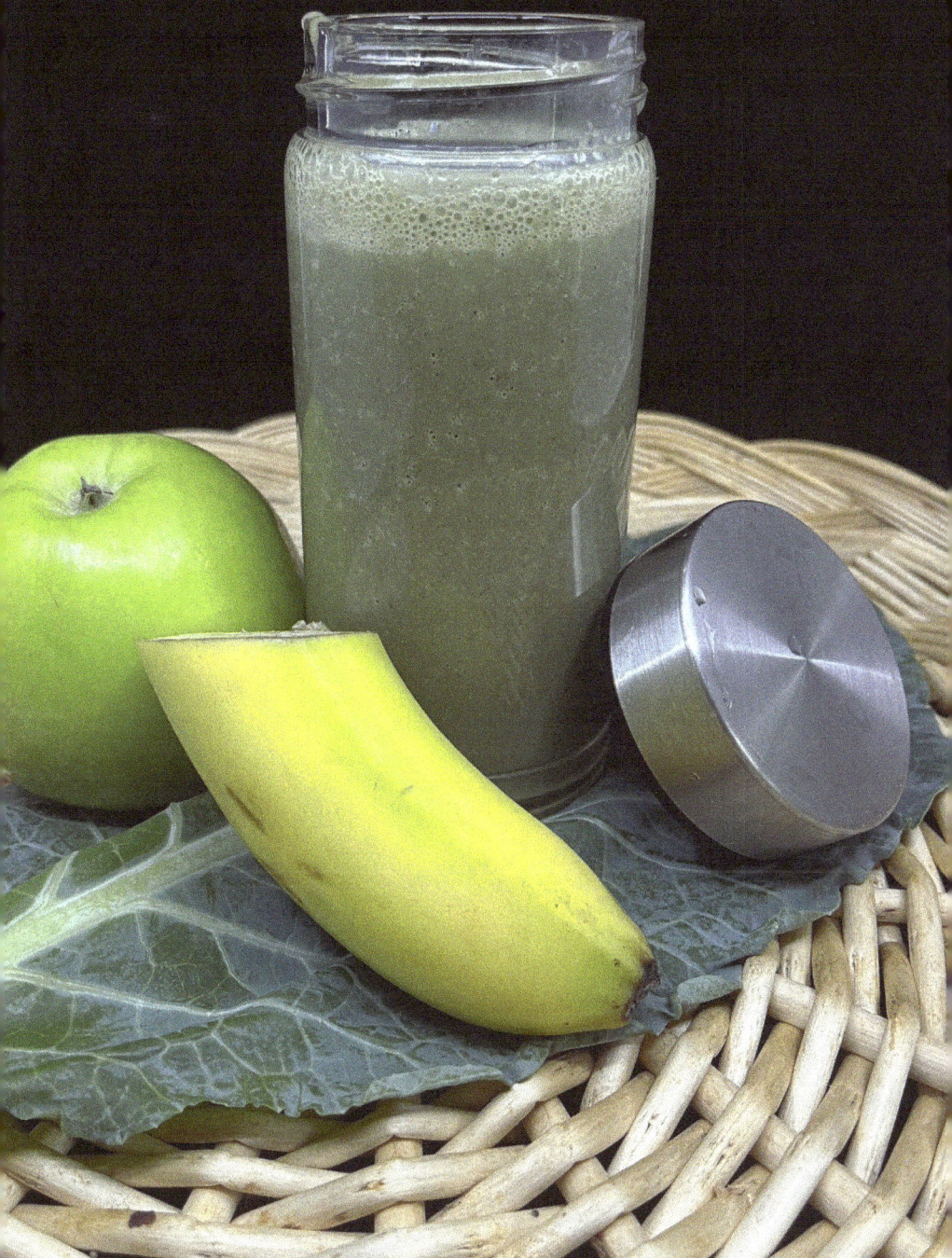

Eternal Youth Green Smoothie

IB2. Eternal Youth Green Smoothie

Discover the magic of collard greens, renowned for their diabetes-fighting prowess. Almond milk, banana, and apple unite in harmony, complemented by a touch of date to provide probiotics and antifungal goodness. And let's not forget the powerful anti-aging benefits of moringa. A deliciously healthy blend awaits you!

INGREDIENTS

(Serves 1)

» 1 green apple
» ½ banana
» 1 cup collard greens (1 ½ large leaves makes approximate 1 cup) or spinach or kale
» 2 tablespoons peanut butter or sunflower butter
» 1 tablespoon flaxseed
» 1 tablespoon of moringa powder
» 1 cup almond milk or water
» 5 ice cubes
» Alternative: 1 tablespoon honey or 1 date (for sweetness)

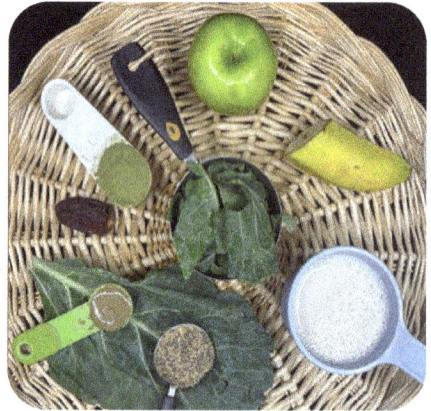

INSTRUCTIONS

1. Place all ingredients in the blender and blend until smooth. BON APPETITE!

Eternal Youth Green Smoothie's Ingredients

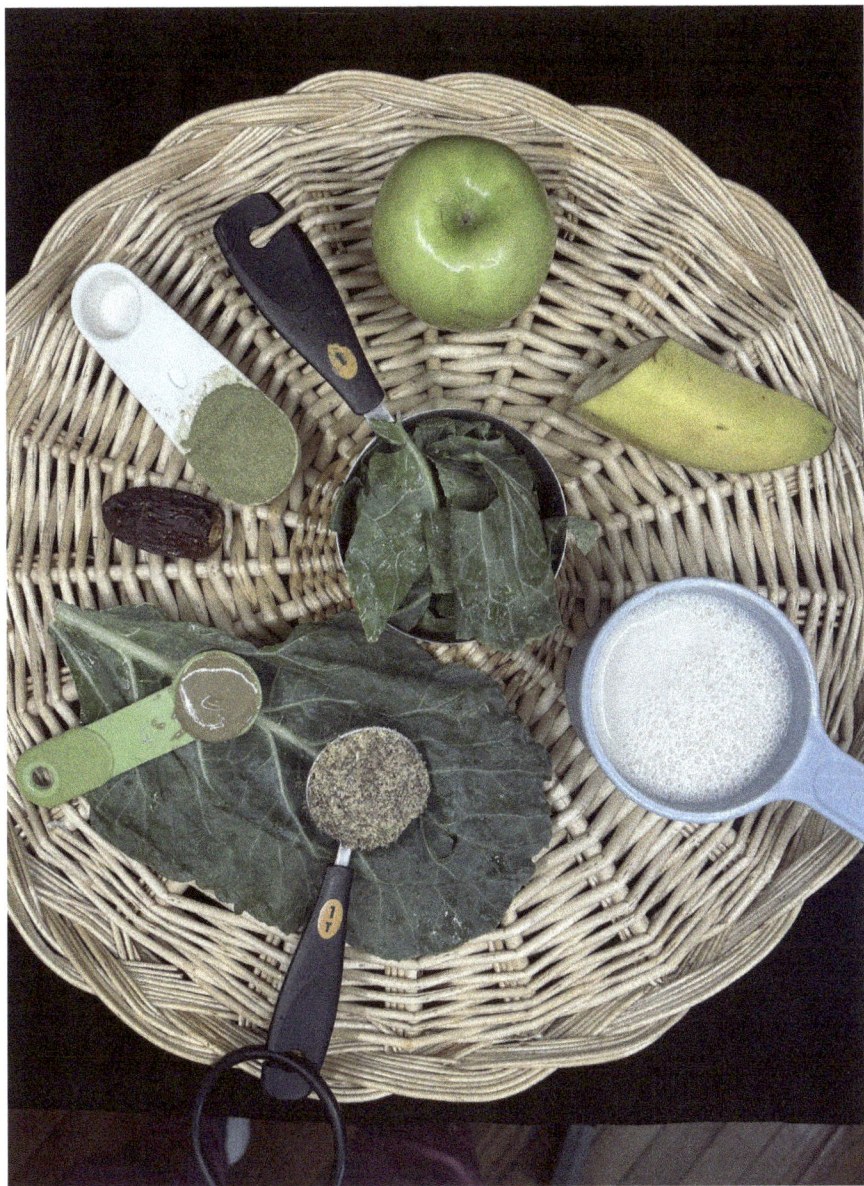

Eternal Youth Green nutrition facts and benefits

NUTRITION FACTS
(1 serving)

Calories: 255kcal
Carbohydrates: 34g
Protein: 7.5g
Fat: 12g
Saturated Fat: 1.5g
Cholesterol: 0mg
Sodium: 252mg
Potassium: 534mg
Fiber: 6g
Sugar: 20g

HEALTH BENEFITS: Spinach packs high amounts of antioxidants, which can also help to fight cancer [23]. Zeaxanthin and lutein in spinach work to prevent macular degeneration and cataracts, which are major causes of blindness [24]. A nutrient that also occurs in many plant foods (quercetin) may offer anti-inflammatory, antiviral, anticancer, and antidepressant effects, according to animal studies [9]. Flaxseed is particularly high in thiamine, a B vitamin that plays a key role in energy metabolism as well as cell function. It's also a great source of copper, which is involved in brain development, immune health, and iron metabolism [30]. Collard greens possess a beneficial effect against diabetes and can be used in the program diet of diabetic patients [31]. Dates come with antifungal, probiotic, and antioxidant functional properties [32]. Consumption of moringa leaves has the potential to improve hemoglobin and serum retinol levels and should be encouraged as part of a regular diet [33]. Moringa oleifera (M. oleifera), widely used in tropical and subtropical regions, has also been reported to possess good anti-aging benefits on skincare [34].

Frozen Food or Fresh Food?

Choice: It depends.

Some researchers have found that in the case of frozen mushrooms, results showed that edible mushrooms have a higher content of bio elements that are easily bio accessible, which indicates their health-promoting properties [35]. However, other researchers that analyzed Broccoli, cauliflower, corn, green beans, green peas, spinach, blueberries, and strawberries found that they do not support the common belief of consumers that fresh food comes with significantly greater nutritional value than their frozen counterparts [36].

Ginger – Pealed or Unpeeled?

Researchers in Germany found that unpeeled ginger exhibited more intense citrus-like and fresh impressions compared to peeled ginger. Unpeeled ginger contained a higher total of polyphenol (84.49 mg/100 g) in comparison with peeled ginger (76.53 mg/100 g and 28.6 g/kg)[37]. Moreover, the industrial use of ginger after peeling results in large amounts of agro-waste.

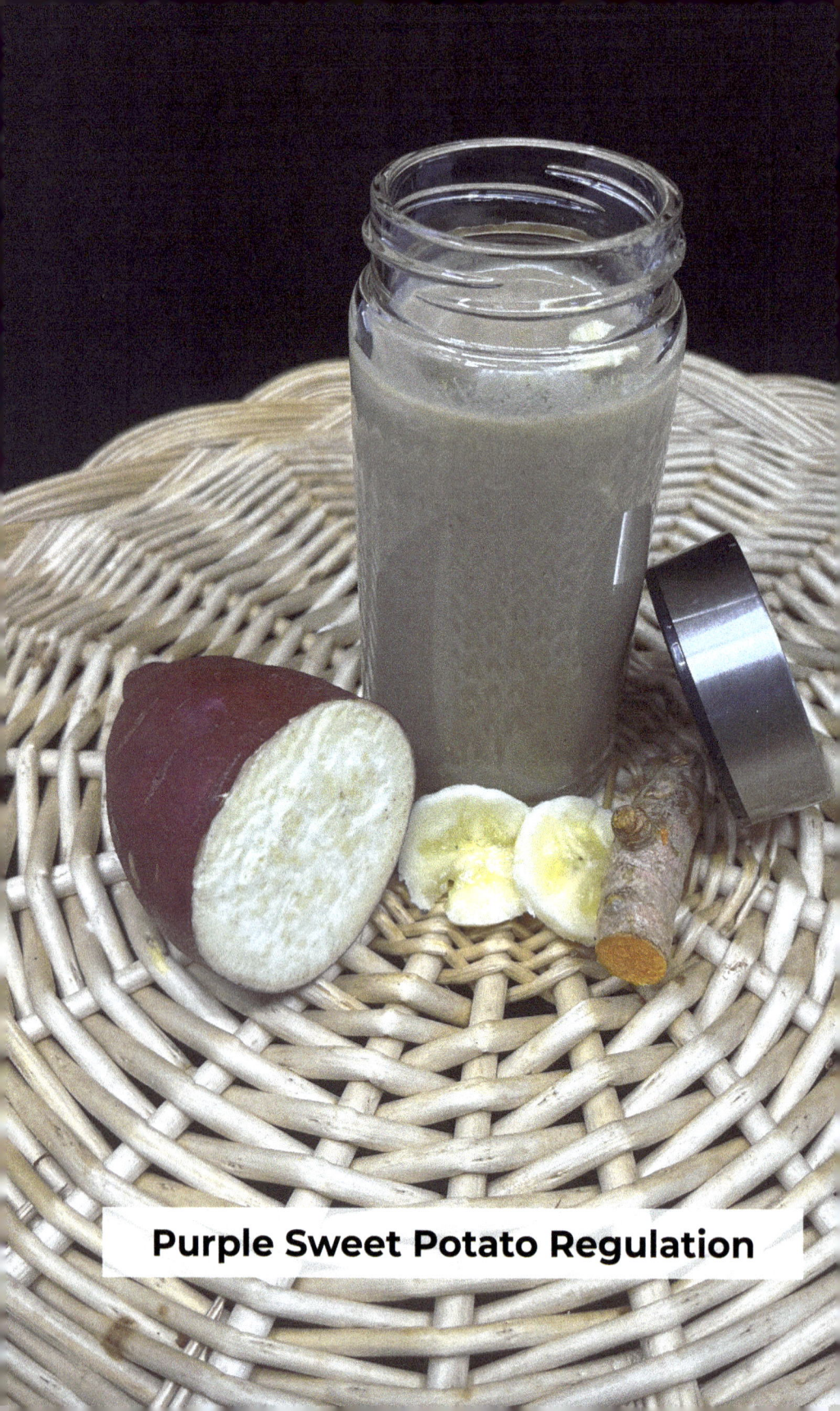

Purple Sweet Potato Regulation

IB3. Purple Sweet Potato Regulation

Backed by research for its immune-modulating effects, this smoothie features maca and healing manuka honey for a powerful punch. Banana brings antioxidant, anti-diabetic, and anti-inflammatory benefits, making this smoothie a true powerhouse of wellness.

INGREDIENTS

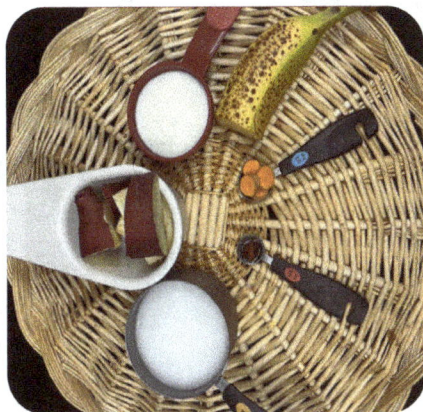

🛎 (Serves 1)

» 1 cup raw purple sweet potato with the skin on (if you can't stand the flavor of raw sweet potato, boil it for 5 minutes)
» 1/2 banana
» 1/2 teaspoon of turmeric (curcuma)
» A pinch of black pepper
» ½ teaspoon vanilla extract
» 1 cup of coconut water or filtered water
» 1/2 cup plain cultured low-fat milk probiotic (kefir) or cultured oat milk (contains probiotic)
» ½ cup of filtered water and 1/3 cup of ice cubes (5 ice cubes)
» 1 teaspoon of manuka honey or raw honey (optional)

INSTRUCTIONS

1. Add all of the ingredients (apart from the water) to a blender.
2. Then pour in the 1/2 cup of water plus 1/3 cup of ice cubes and blend on the highest setting until smooth. If the drink is too thick, add another ½ cup of water and pulse a few times.
3. Taste for sweetness and add sugar free honey or dates.

Purple Sweet Potato Regulation's Ingredients

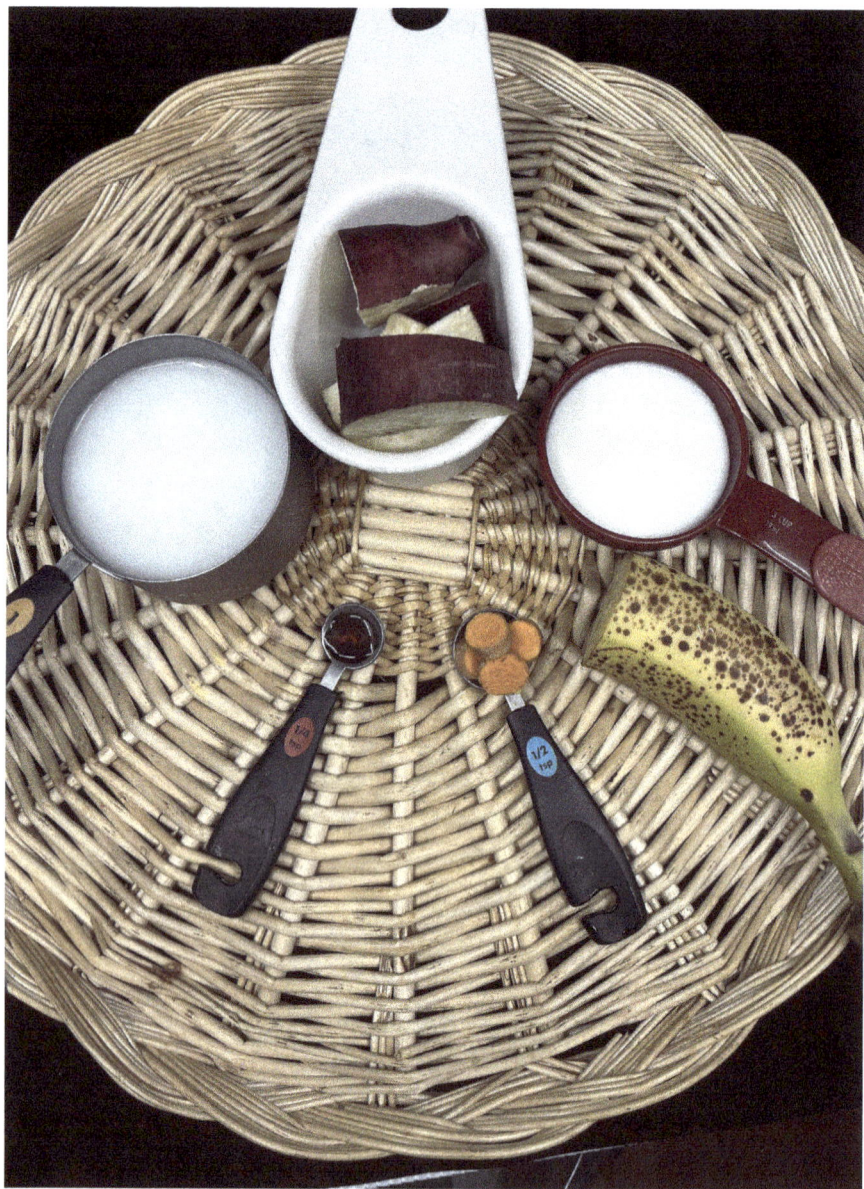

Purple Sweet Potato Regulation nutrition facts and benefits

NUTRITION FACTS (per serving)

Calories: 125 kcal
Carbohydrates: 30 g
Protein: 4.5 g
Fat: 0g
Saturated Fat: 0 g
Cholesterol: 0 mg
Sodium: 0 mg
Potassium: 600 mg
Fiber: 3 g
Sugar: 8 g
Vitamin C: 22

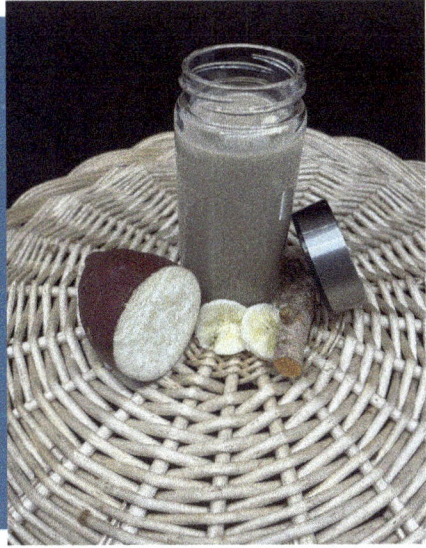

HEALTH BENEFITS: Curcumin, a bioactive substance found in turmeric, has been shown to possess anti-inflammatory properties [25]. Both Curcuma (turmeric) and purple sweet potato (when used together) have demonstrated positive effects on immunomodulation [38]. Purple sweet potato has also been associated with a potential metabolomic mechanism that regulates intestinal inflammation [39]. Manuka honey has the potential to support immune homeostasis by enhancing microbial sensing through mucosal-associated invariant T cells [41]. Moreover, the components present in manuka honey have shown the ability to induce cytokine production, which could potentially lead to the development of novel therapies for improving wound healing in patients with acute and chronic wounds [42]. Banana contains various bioactive compounds, such as alkaloids, phenols, flavonoids, tannins, and saponins, with reported therapeutic benefits that include antioxidant, anti-diabetic, anti-cancer, anti-inflammatory, and anti-microbial activities [43]. Vanilla is rich in antioxidants. Cultured low fat milk or plant-based contains probiotics, and dates are rich in fiber and antioxidants.

IB4. Healing Juices using a Juice Extractor.

I present two exquisite, anti-inflammatory super juices that have been lovingly prepared for my family's well-being. Crafting these nutritional elixirs is a labor of love, requiring approximately half an hour of dedication, from meticulously washing the freshest ingredients to thoroughly cleaning the juice extractor. The effort is truly worth it, as I make these nourishing blends every other day, ensuring a constant supply of healthful goodness.

To preserve the integrity of the juices, I store them in glass containers, ready to be savored over the next few days. To relish the maximum benefits of these concoctions, it's ideal to consume them within 48 hours, allowing the vibrant array of nutrients and antioxidants to work wonders for your body. Embrace the joy of wellness with every sip, as these super juices pave the way to a healthier and more vibrant life.

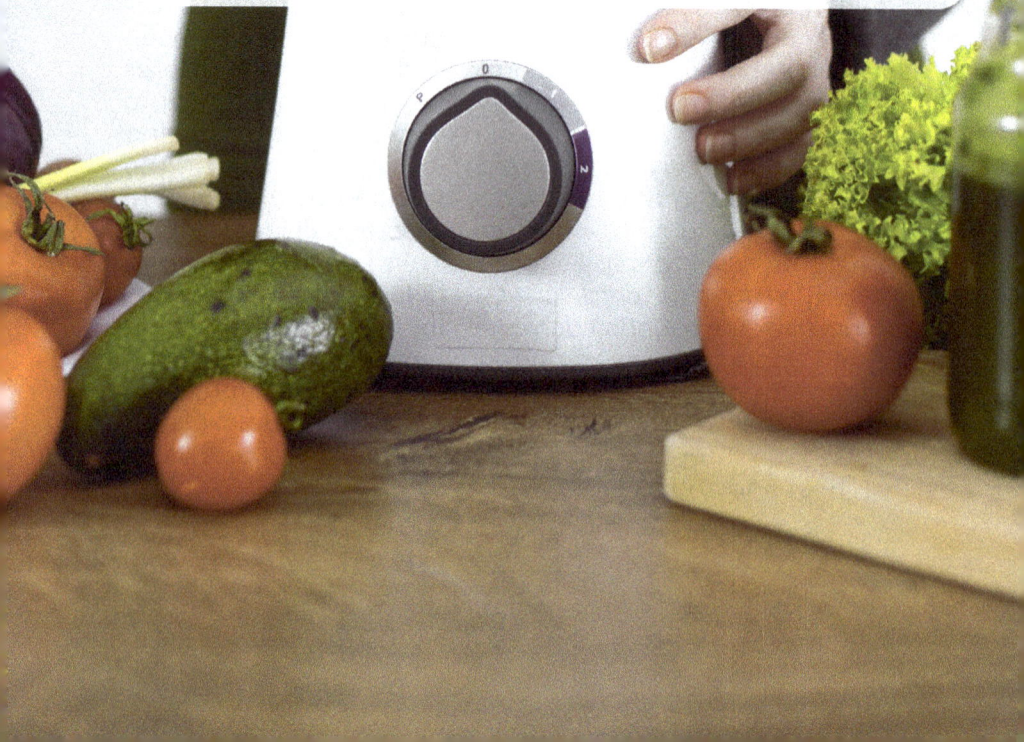

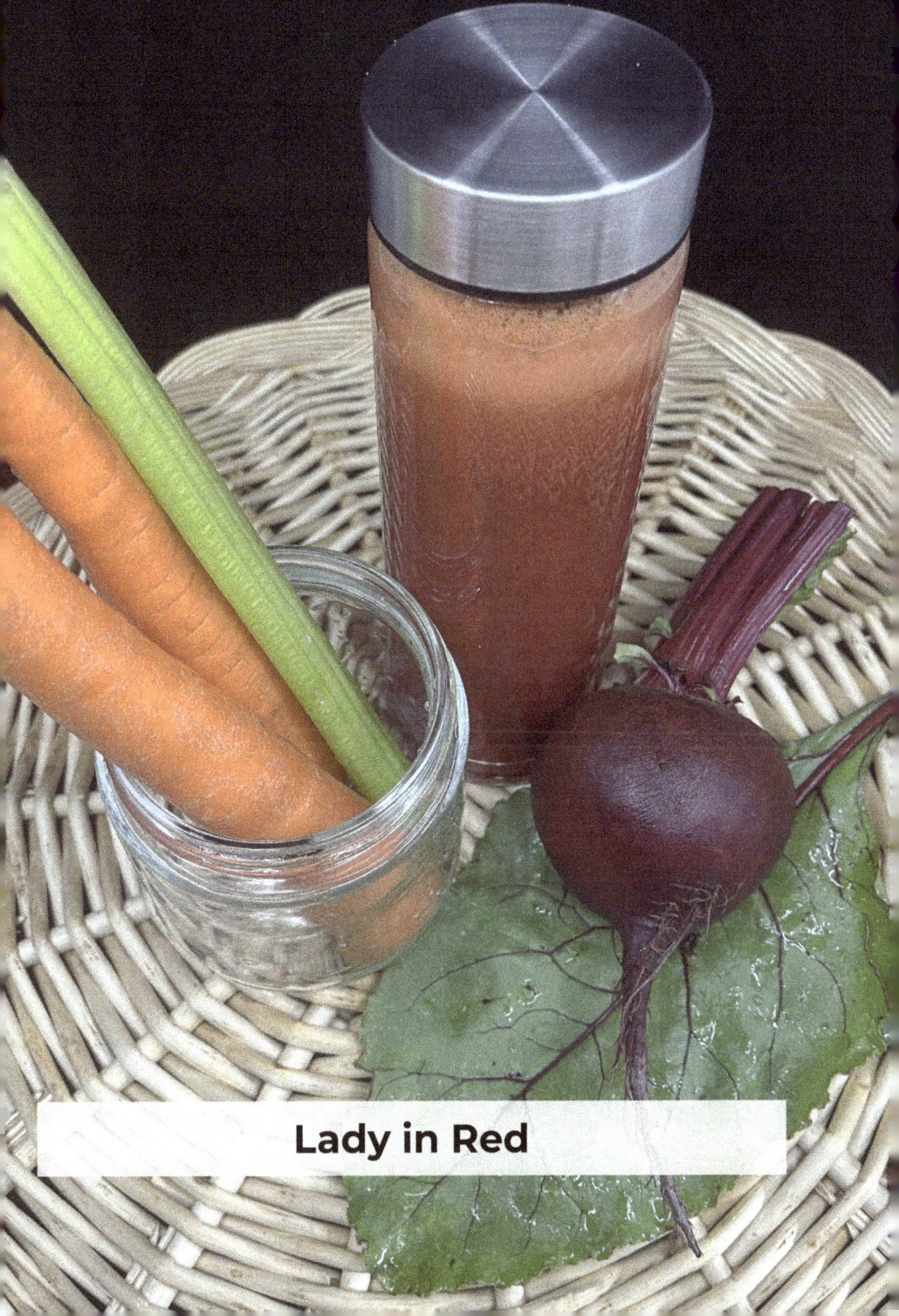
Lady in Red

IB41. Lady in Red

Indulge in the invigorating "Lady in Red" juice, boasting beetroots, carrots, celery, and green apples, spiced with turmeric and ginger. Black pepper and cinnamon provide extra antioxidants. Enjoy the probiotic benefits of vegetable juices, while celery aids in combating obesity. Elevate your health with this flavorful and nutrient-packed delight!

INGREDIENTS

(Serves 5)

For this juice recipe, you will need the following ingredients:
» 15 medium unpeeled carrots
» 2 medium unpeeled beet-roots
» 6 beet leaves (optional)
» 6 celery sticks
» 2 medium green apples (seeds removed)
» ¼ cup turmeric chunks
» 1/3 cup ginger chunks
» 1 teaspoon cinnamon
» ½ teaspoon black pepper
» 1 small citrus fruit (mandarin, tangerine, or orange) including the peel (optional)

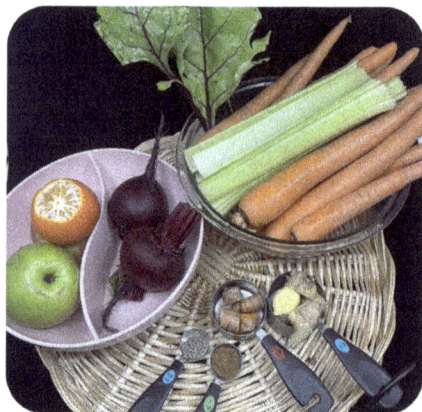

INSTRUCTIONS

1. To prepare the juice, cut the carrots, beetroots, celery, apples, turmeric, ginger, and citrus fruit (if using) into chunks suitable for your juicer. Place all the ingredients into the extractor and then extract the juice. Once the juice is ready, you can add the cinnamon and black pepper to the final product. Mix it well using a large spoon. If you prefer, you can also include the beet leaves for added nutrition.

2. It is recommended to drink the juice immediately after preparation to enjoy its freshness and nutritional benefits. However, if you are not planning to consume it right away, pour it into glass containers with lids and store them in the refrigerator. Remember to consume the juice within the next 48 hours for optimal taste and quality.

Lady in Red nutrition facts and benefits

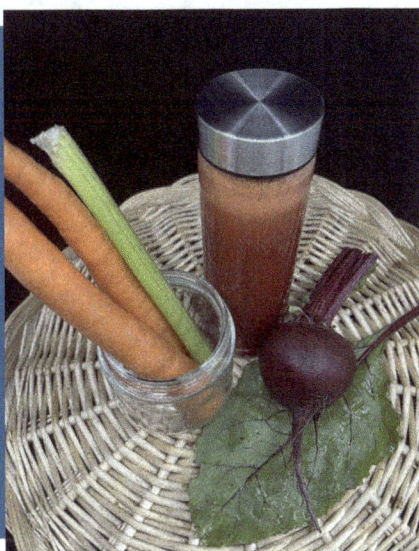

NUTRITION FACTS (1 serving)

Calories: 210kcal
Carbohydrates: 12g
Protein: 4g
Fat: 8g
Saturated Fat: 0g
Cholesterol: 0mg
Sodium: 21mg
Potassium: 21mg
Fiber: 10g
Sugar: 6.3g

HEALTH BENEFITS: The vegetables used for this juice (carrot, beetroot) consist of a high number of antioxidants like carotenoids in carrot, betaxanthins and betacyanins in beetroot [44]. These antioxidants provide numerous health benefits for the human body. The three bacterial strains Lactobacillus plantarum, and Lactobacillus delbrueckii used in three types of juices including carrot juice and beetroot juice showed good growth for probiotics. Vegetable juices also have almost zero fat content and are high in fiber, meaning that people on a low fat free diet can consume this product [44]. Studies have found that enzyme-treated celery extract has an anti-obesity effect [45].

Lady in Red's Ingredients

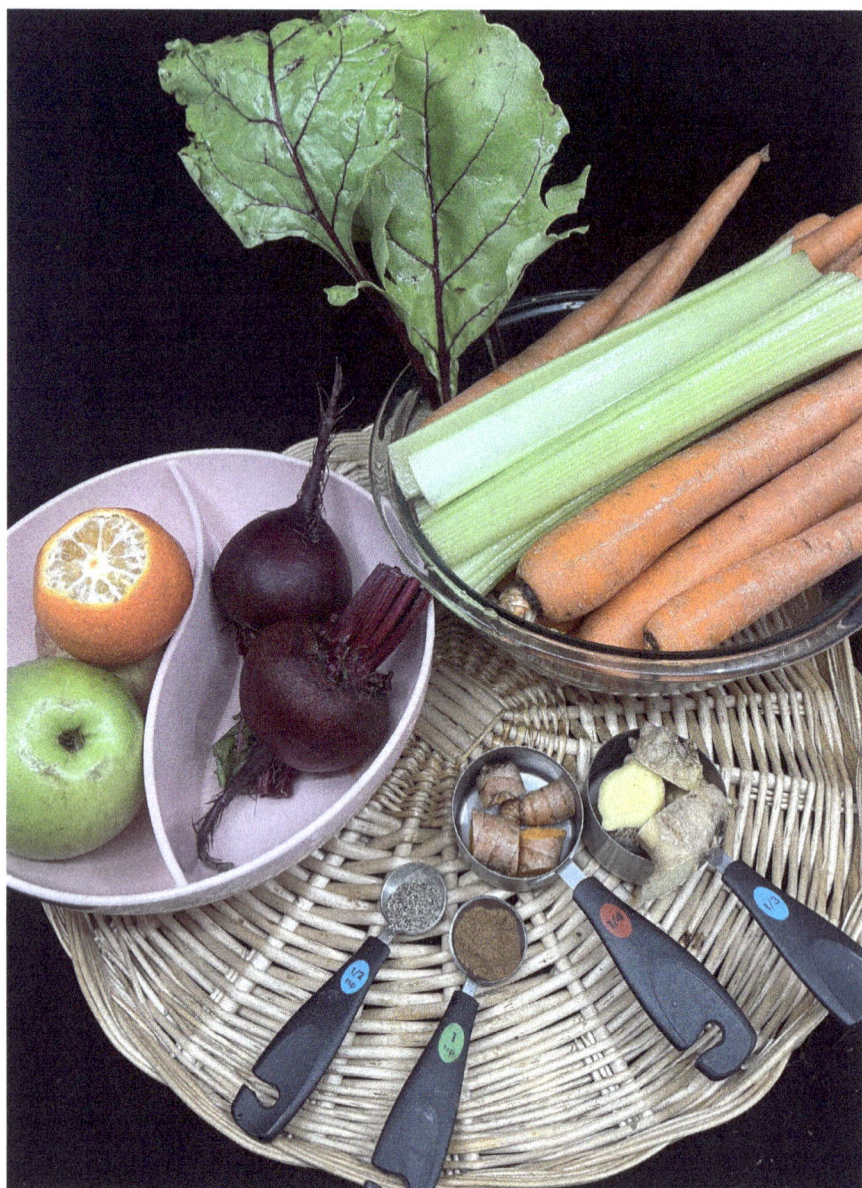

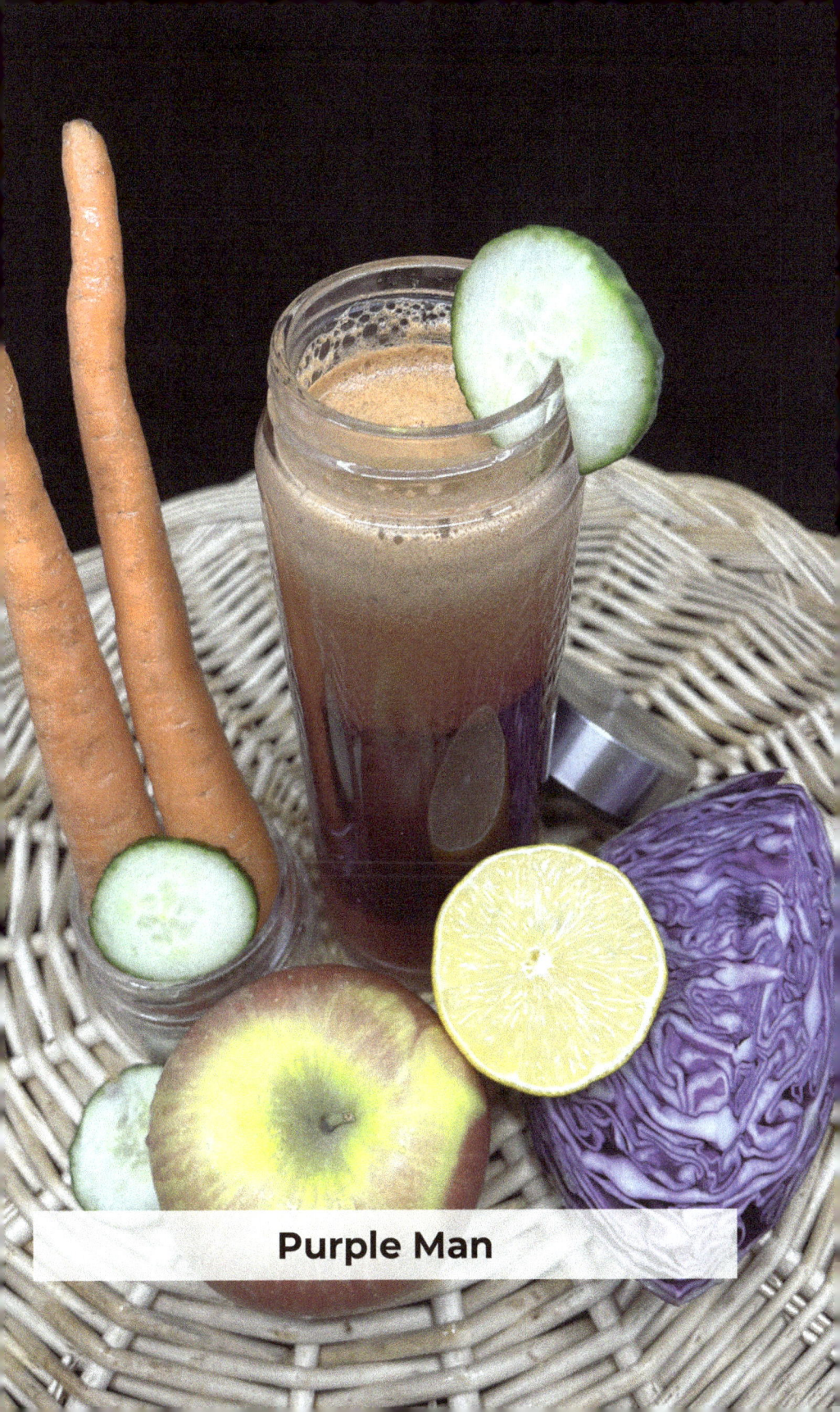
Purple Man

IB42. Purple Man

Discover the mighty "Purple Man" vegetable juice. Brimming with antioxidants from carrots, purple cabbage, and cucumber, it serves to nourish a healthy gut microbiota. Ginger and curcumin unite to combat inflammation, while lemon offers antimicrobial benefits. Apples contribute their potent polyphenols, safeguarding against environmental damage. Sip your way to vitality with this nutrient-packed elixir!

INGREDIENTS

🍽 **(Serves 5)**

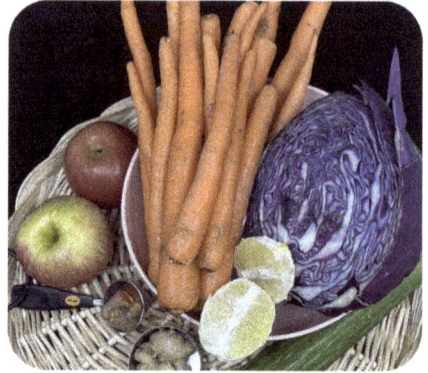

For this juice recipe, you will need the following ingredients:
» 15 medium unpeeled carrots
» ½ red cabbage (known as purple)
» 1 large cucumber
» 2 medium unpeeled apples (seeds removed)
» 1 tablespoon of turmeric chunks
» 1/3 cup of ginger chunks
» 1 lemon, peeled (seeds removed)
» 1 teaspoon of cinnamon
» ½ teaspoon of black pepper

INSTRUCTIONS

1. To prepare the juice, cut the carrots, red cabbage, cucumber, apples, turmeric, ginger, and lemon into chunks suitable for your juicer. Place all the ingredients into the extractor and proceed to extract the juice. Once the juice has been extracted, add the cinnamon and black pepper to the final product and mix it well using a large spoon. It is recommended to drink the juice immediately after preparation. However, if you are not planning to consume it right away, pour it into glass containers with lids before storing them in the refrigerator. Remember to consume the juice within the next 48 hours for optimal freshness.

Purple Man's Ingredients

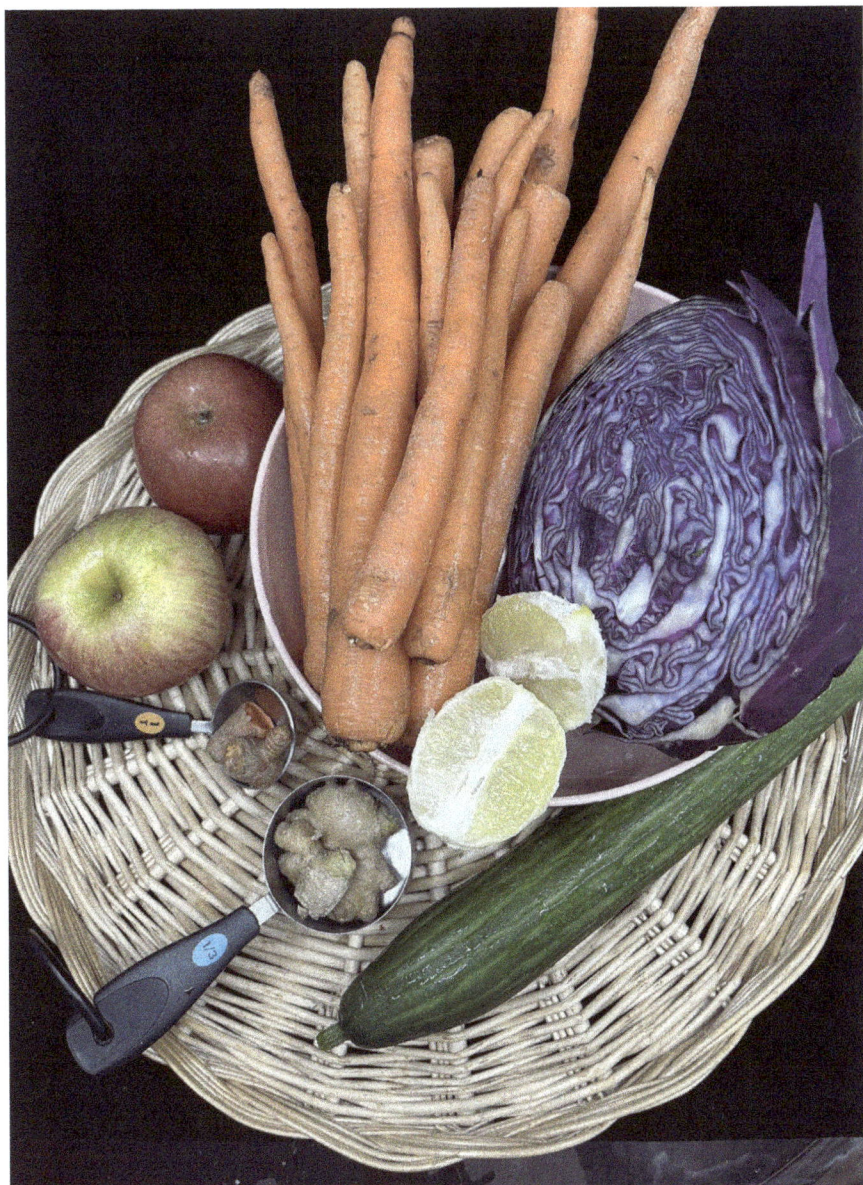

Purple Man nutrition facts and benefits

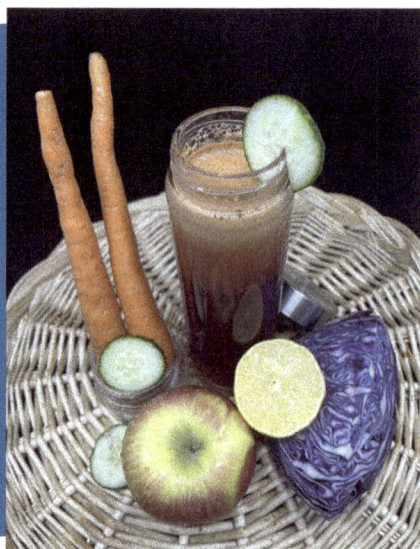

NUTRITION FACTS
(per serving)

Calories: 210 kcal
Carbohydrates: 36g
Protein: 4g
Fat: 8g
Saturated Fat: 1g
Cholesterol: 0mg
Sodium: 183mg
Potassium: 102mg
Fiber: 10g
Sugar: 11g

HEALTH BENEFITS: The vegetables used in juices offer a high number of antioxidants, such as the three bacterial strains Lactobacillus plantarum, and Lactobacillus delbrueckii are commonly found in juices, such as carrot juice. Vegetable juices also have almost zero fat content and are high in fiber, so those on a low fat free diet can safely consume this product [44]. Sulfated polysaccharides from cucumber has been found to modulate the gut microbiota by promoting the growth of probiotics [46]. The color of red cabbage (Brassica oleracea var. capitata) is due to anthocyanin accumulation [47]. Moreover, the number of total anthocyanins in red cabbage was found to correlate positively with the total antioxidant power, thus implicating the potential health benefit of red cabbage to our health [47]. The antifungal efficacy of lemon juice has been confirmed in addition to its actual antimicrobial benefits [48, 49]. Overweight/obese women may benefit from apple or berry juice as part of a healthy lifestyle to improve their lipid profile, and thus, contribute to cardiovascular health [49]. Fruits such as apples are a dietary source of polyphenols and offer a number of health benefits [50].

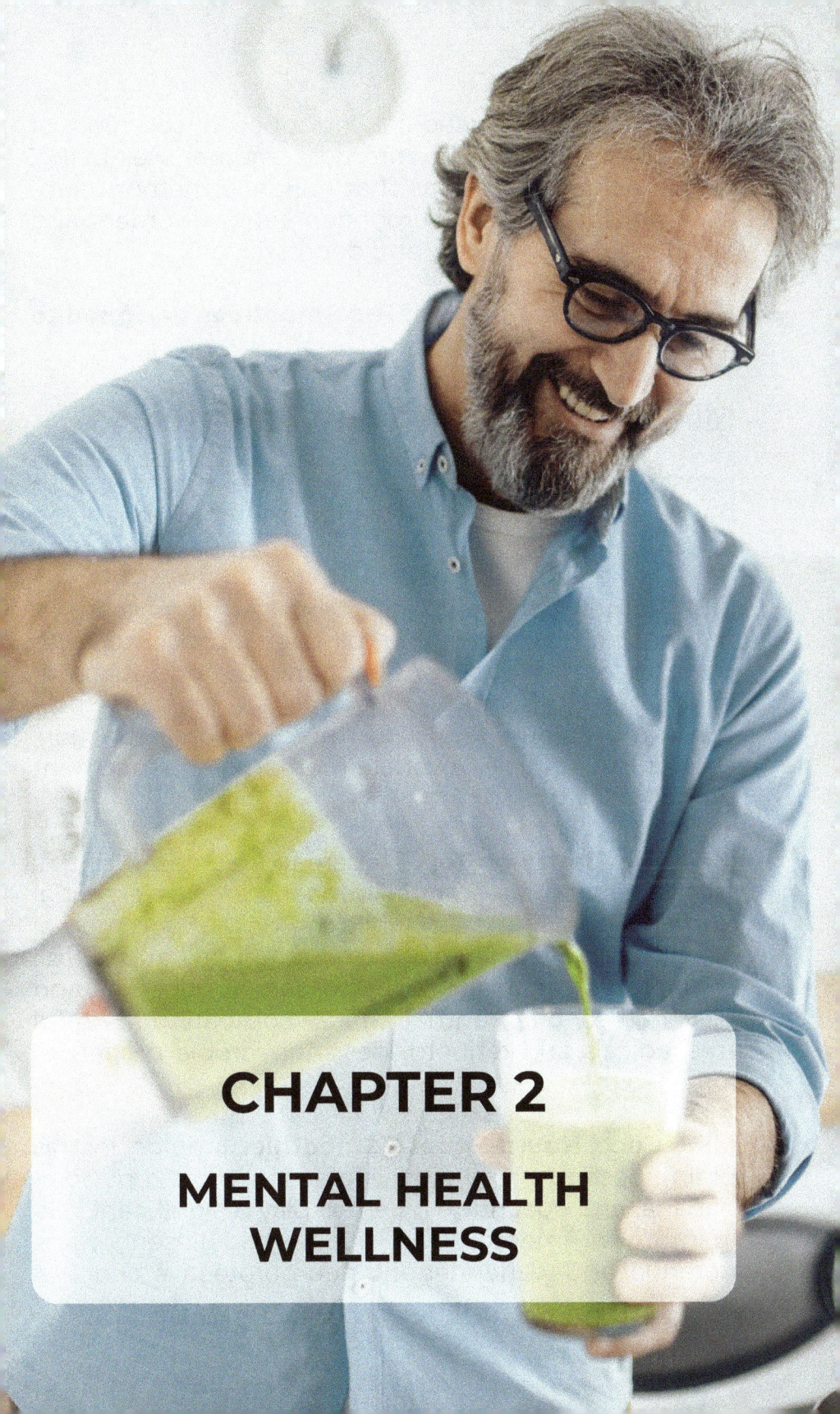

CHAPTER 2

MENTAL HEALTH WELLNESS

In the following section, I introduce a selection of smoothies designed to promote mental well-being. These include smoothies that enhance memory, support individuals with neurodegenerative disorders, and aid in alleviating anxiety and depression.

Below is a description of the Smoothies designed to support Mental Wellness

ME: Memory Enhancing Smoothies

Boost your brainpower and improve memory with my selection of carefully crafted memory-enhancing smoothies:

ME1. **Remember Now!** This delightful blend features nutrient-rich avocado and blueberries, packed with powerful antioxidants. Ashwagandha adds its anti-inflammatory benefits while also enhancing skin condition. Walnuts, known for improving brain function, contribute to the overall memory enhancement properties of this smoothie.

ME2. **The Cherry on Top.** Prepare to be amazed by this fantastic smoothie. Cannellini beans provide essential nutrients for brain health, while cherries support mental alertness. Cloves aid memory retention, and Brazil nuts protect against brain disorders. Blueberries and blackberries offer anthocyanins, combating harmful free radicals, and kefir provides antimicrobial properties for a healthier brain.

ME3. **Coco Neuro-Fitness Smoothie.** Indulge in this brain-boosting blend of kale, ginseng, protein powder, banana, and coconut oil. Berries play a significant role in improving memory and mood, while ginseng offers potential anti-Alzheimer and neuroprotective benefits.

The inclusion of coconut oil directly supports brain power.

ME4. **Apricot Focus Smoothie.** Experience the power of Bacopa monnieri in this smoothie, providing neuroprotective effects against Parkinson's disease. Apricots with lutein help prevent Alzheimer's disease, and carrot juice acts as a neuroprotective factor against neuronal damage.

ND: Smoothies for Neurodegenerative Disorders

Prepare to embark on a transformative journey with my sensational smoothies specifically crafted to support neurodegenerative disorders:

ND1. **Golden Neuro Healer**. Unleash the power of healing with my Golden Neuro Healer smoothie! Fava beans and golden berries join forces to form an invincible shield against Parkinson's disease. Brace yourself for the magic of turmeric, Brazil nuts, and maca as they provide unparalleled brain support, while sunflower seeds and cinnamon work their wonders by reducing inflammation and managing diabetes. Get ready to feel the vitality coursing through your body!

ND2. **Purple Brain Detox.** Get ready to defy aging and embrace cognitive brilliance with my purple Brain Detox smoothie! Watch as blueberries work their magic, reversing age-related cognitive deficits, while strawberries unleash their antioxidant prowess. Turmeric takes center stage as it disrupts the toxic loop responsible for Parkinson's disease. Meanwhile, the dynamic duo of coconut milk and water comes to the rescue by suppressing inflammatory responses. And let's not forget the pecans, adding their touch of perfection in preventing obesity. Experience a rejuvenation like never before!

ND3. **Kudos Kiwi Neurotransmitter.** Prepare for an explosion of neurotransmitter support with my Kudos Kiwi Neurotransmitter smoothie! Kiwis, dates, and turmeric unite to create an unbeatable combination in the fight against neurodegenerative disorders. Chia, pineapple, and hemp seeds come to the rescue by preventing inflammation and promoting optimal brain health. This smoothie is a celebration of life and vitality!

ND4. **No Brainer Clementine.** Simplicity meets power in my No Brainer Clementine smoothie! Clementine, banana, turmeric, and coconut milk come together to form a forceful blend designed to combat brain cell-damaging diseases like Parkinson's, Alzheimer's, and dementia. Embrace the magic of these ingredients as they work harmoniously to invigorate your mind and protect your precious memories.

Get ready to witness the extraordinary impact of these smoothies as they take your health and well-being to new heights. Each sip is a step towards a brighter and more vibrant future!

MH: Smoothies to reduce anxiety and depression.

Get ready to experience a burst of excitement with tantalizing, mood-boosting smoothies:

MH1. **Relax, Psych Biotic Pomegranate!** Indulge in the ultimate relaxation with this sensational smoothie! I've combined probiotics from cultured oat milk and prebiotics from rolled oats to create a neuroprotective psych biotic effect that will leave you feeling invigorated.

But that's not all – the magic of pomegranate will whisk away your worries as it moderates anxiety. And brace yourself for the incredible benefits of Brazil nuts and ginseng, delivering a powerhouse of neuroprotective properties that will soon have you beaming with joy!

MH2. **A Peaceful Date.** Prepare to embark on a journey of tranquility with this blissful smoothie! Almonds and dates team up to support memory while melting away anxiety and depression, leaving you with a sense of serenity. But that's not all – the delightful touch of maca and rolled oats adds an extra dose of calm to your mind, creating a peaceful oasis you won't ever want to leave.

MH3. **Chocolate Chill Out.** It's time to treat yourself to pure bliss with our Chocolate Chill Out smoothie! Take pleasure in the exquisite flavors of figs, banana, and cacao, while your brain revels in their brain-boosting benefits. And here's the secret ingredient: maca, which unleashes its natural antidepressant effects to uplift your spirits and leave you floating on cloud nine!

MH4. **The Pear of My Eye.** Feel the love with The Pear of My Eye smoothie! Dive into a luscious blend of coconut water, pear, mango, matcha, and hemp hearts that will instantly whisk you away to a tranquil paradise. This enchanting concoction provides essential nutrients that not only manage stress but also promote a profound sense of calm and well-being, making it your new favorite soul-soother.

Experience the thrill of these exciting smoothies as they take your taste buds and mind on an unforgettable adventure of flavor and nourishment. Get ready to sip your way to pure bliss!

SHOPPING LIST TO SUPPORT MENTAL HEALTH WELLNESS

Berries: Blueberries, strawberries, golden berries, cherries

Fruits: Banana, pineapple, mango, kiwi, avocado, clementine, pomegranate, pear

Greens: Spinach

Roots: Turmeric, ginseng

Additives: Maca powder, cinnamon, chia seeds, ashwagandha, sunflower butter, hemp hearts, matcha powder

Liquid: Almond milk, coconut water, yogurt alternative, cultured low-fat milk (probiotic kefir) or cultured oat milk

Nuts: Almond, walnuts, Brazil nuts, pecans

Others: Cinnamon, black pepper, lemon juice, clove, sea salt

Sweeteners: Raw honey or manuka honey, dates

Source of proteins: Cannellini beans, fava beans, rolled oats.

MEMORY ENHANCING SMOOTHIES

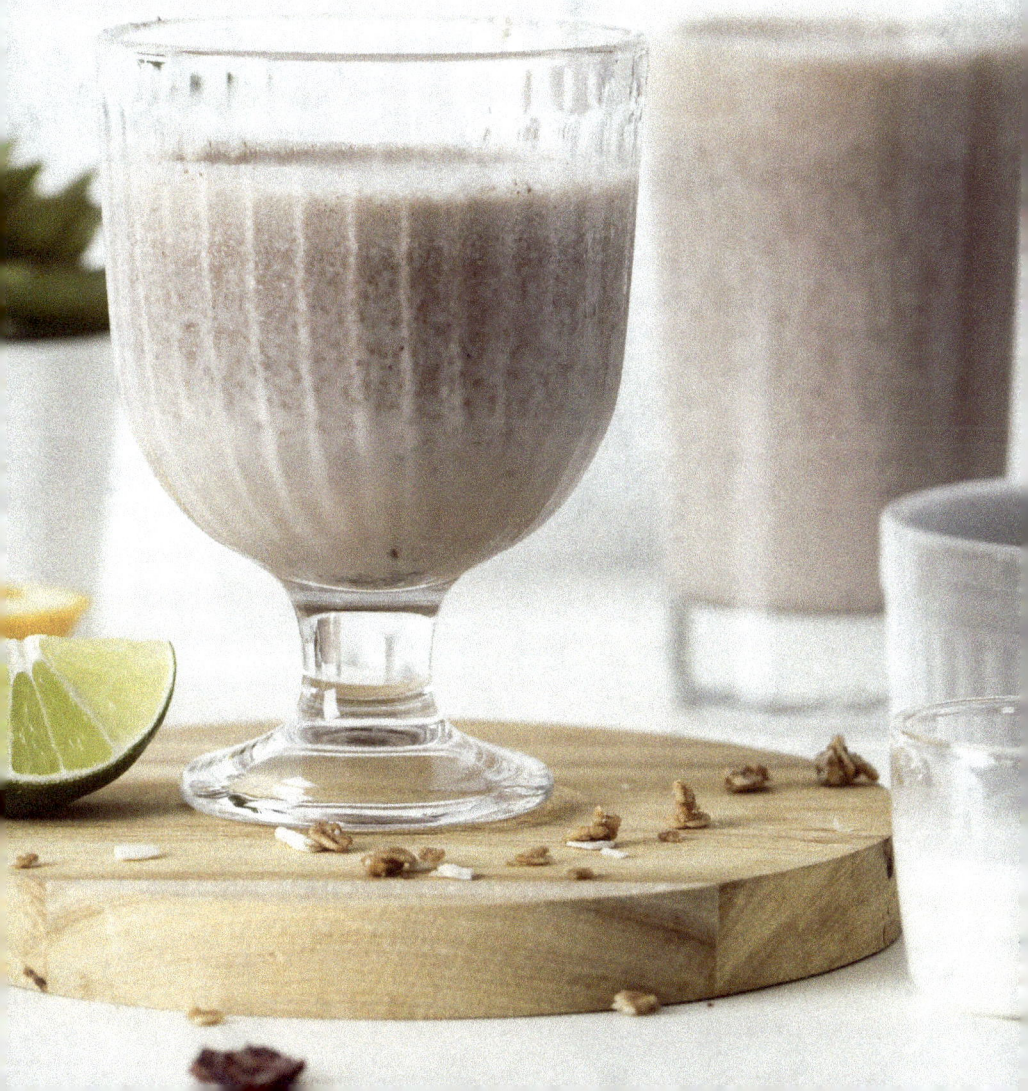

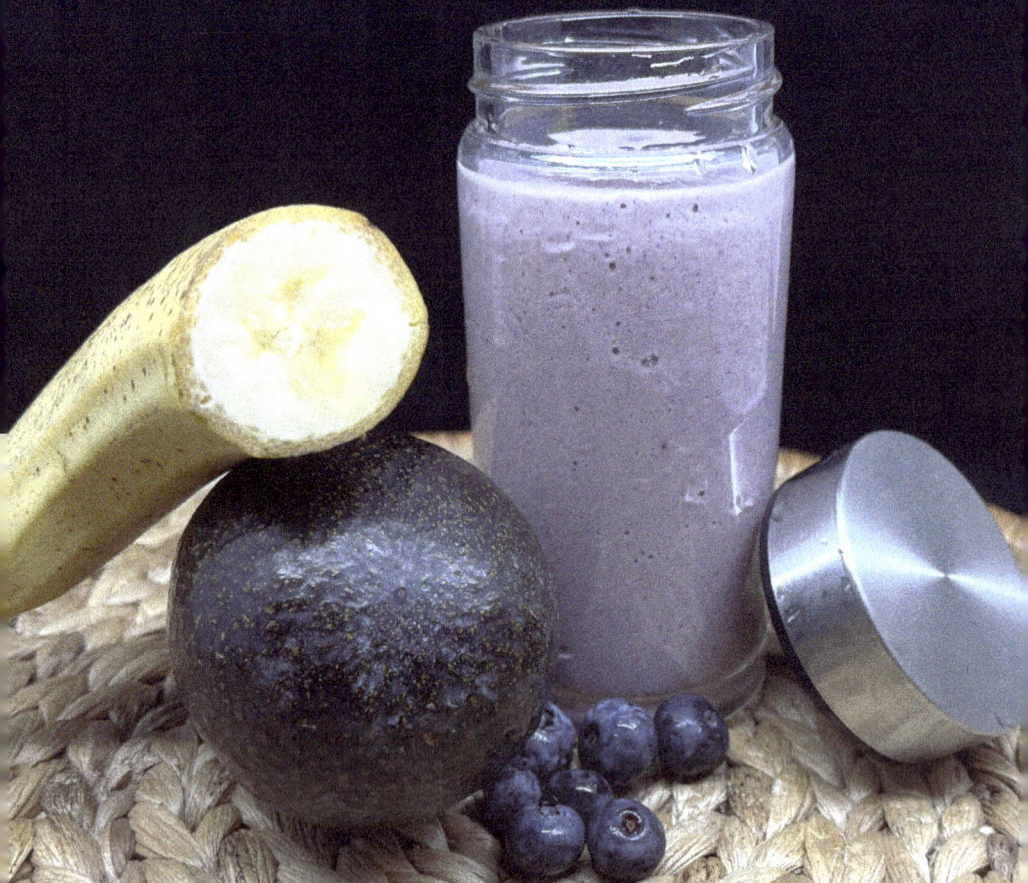

Remember Now!

ME1. Remember Now!

Abundant in powerful antioxidants, allow yourself to indulge in this delightful blend of nutrient-rich avocado and blueberries. Ashwagandha steps up to add its anti-inflammatory benefits while improving skin conditions. With brain-boosting walnuts adding to the memory enhancement properties, this smoothie is a true powerhouse for both the body and mind. Savor the goodness in every sip!

INGREDIENTS

(Serves 1)

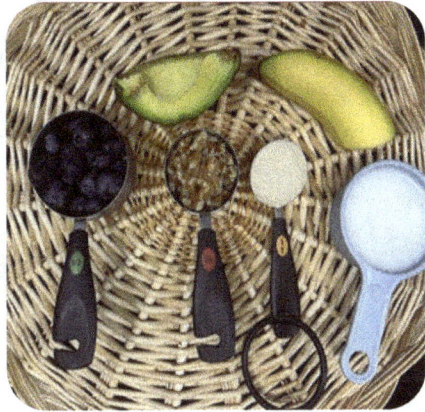

» 1/4 avocado
» 1/2 medium banana
» 1/2 cup blueberries
» 1 tablespoon ashwagandha powder
» 1/2 cup coconut water (or plant-based milk)
» 1/3 cup walnuts (5-6 walnuts)
» Suggestion: add a date and 5 ice cubes

INSTRUCTIONS

1. Add the avocado, blueberries, banana, and ashwagandha powder to your blender.
2. Next, add coconut water (or plant-based milk) and blend everything until smooth.
3. Add your walnuts at the end and then blend for an extra 30 seconds to 1 minute until creamy and smooth. Enjoy!
4. BON APPETITE!

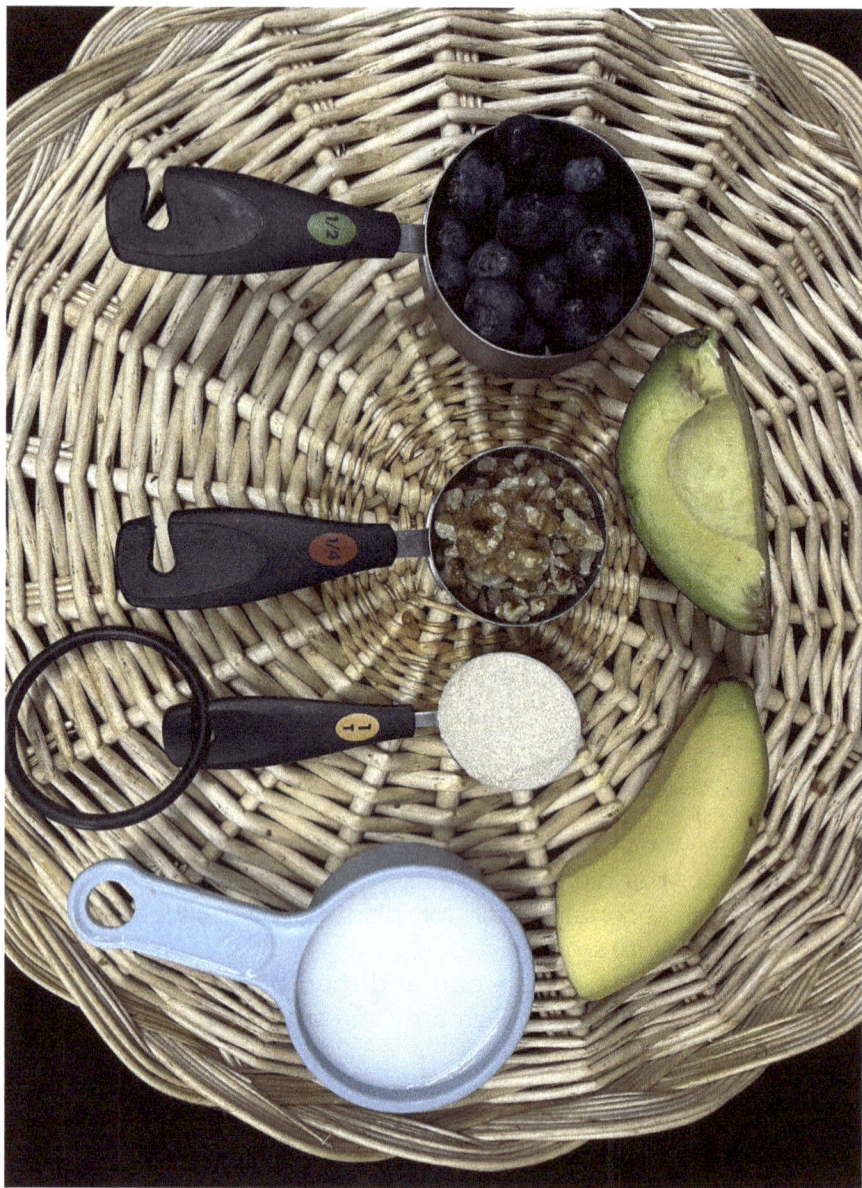

Remember Now! nutrition facts and benefits.

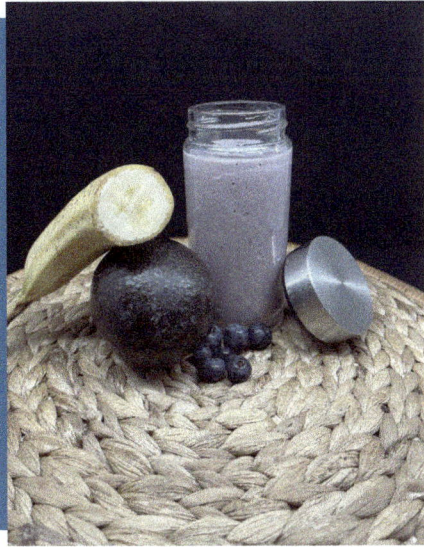

NUTRITION FACTS (1 serving)

Calories: 597kcal
Carbohydrates: 41g
Protein: 30g
Fat: 38g
Saturated Fat: 5g
Cholesterol: 61mg
Sodium: 70mg
Potassium: 1068mg
Fiber: 12g
Sugar: 17g

HEALTH BENEFITS: The antioxidant content of blueberries is thought to be among the highest of all commonly consumed fruits and vegetables. The most significant part of blueberries' health advantages is played by anthocyanins [51]. With greater dietary intake and higher blood levels of antioxidants contained within avocados, such as vitamin C and carotenoids, they have been associated with better cognitive function, improved heart health, and much more [52]. Nutrients found in walnuts may help prevent inflammation from harming your brain and support healthy brain function as you age. Eating walnuts has been associated with improved brain function in older persons, including quicker processing times, greater mental flexibility, and improved memory [53]. Ashwagandha offers antioxidants and anti-inflammatory capabilities in addition to its standardized root extract improving skin condition and the quality of life in photoaged, healthy individuals [54, 55]. Coconut water contains numerous medicinal properties such as antibacterial, antifungal, antiviral, antiparasitic, antidermatophytic, antioxidant, hypoglycemic, hepatoprotective, and immunostimulant [56].

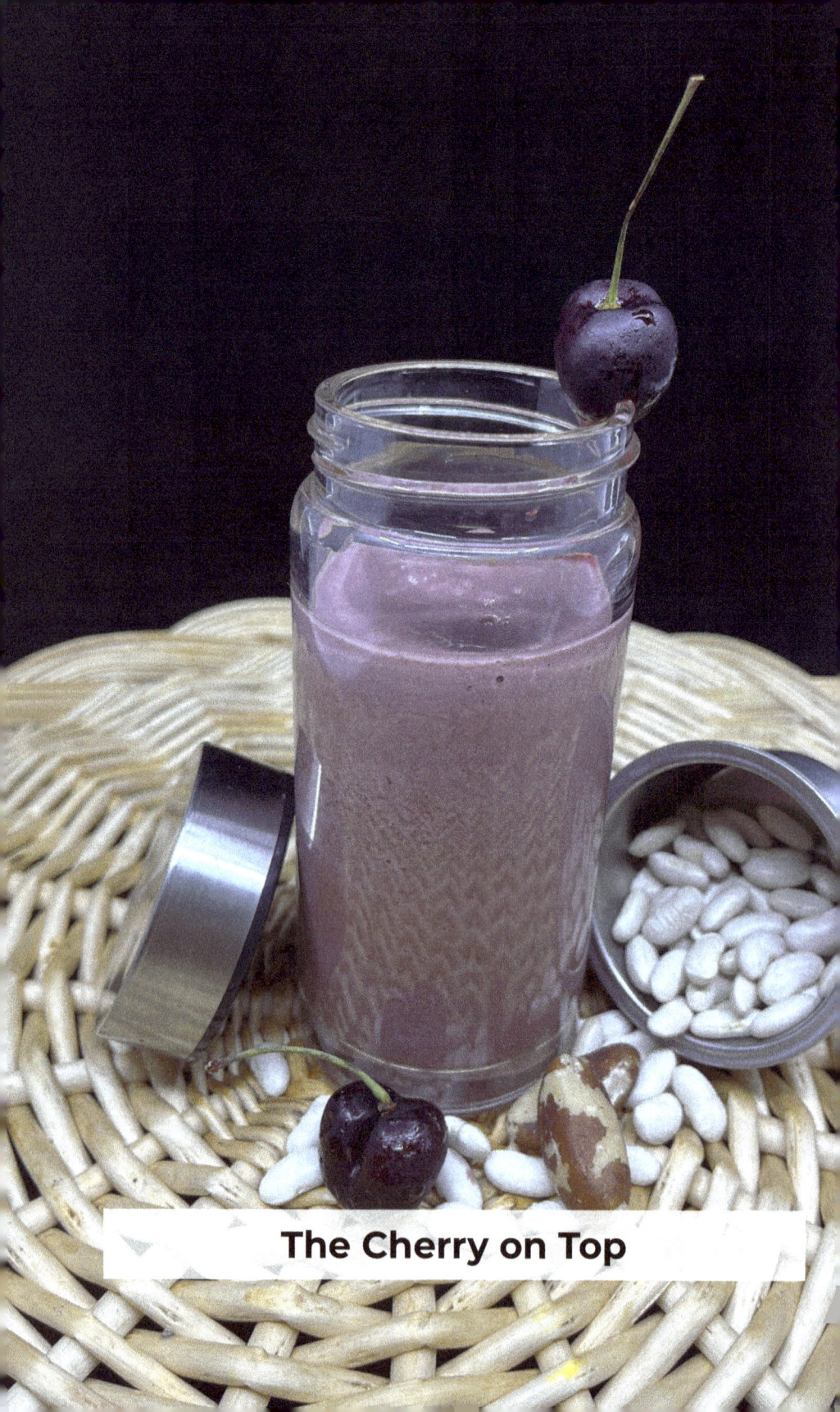

The Cherry on Top

ME2. The Cherry on Top

Get ready to be amazed by this fantastic smoothie! Cannellini beans nurture brain health with essential nutrients, while cherries boost mental alertness. Cloves aid memory retention, and Brazil nuts safeguard against brain disorders. Blueberries and blackberries combat harmful free radicals with their anthocyanins. Meanwhile, kefir contributes its antimicrobial properties to promote a healthier brain. A blend of brain-boosting wonders awaits you!

INGREDIENTS

(Serves 2)

Pre-preparation

» ¼ cannellini beans (after preparation, it will expand to ½ cup)
» 1 cinnamon stick
» 1 clove

Smoothie Preparation

» 1/2 cup boiled cannellini beans (from the pre-preparation stage) or drained and rinsed BPA-free canned cannellini beans (NOTE: While no cooking is required for the addition of beans, simply omit this ingredient if you prefer to keep this smoothie 100% raw.)
» 2 raw Brazil nuts
» 1 cup fresh or frozen cherries
» 1/2 cup fresh or frozen blackberries or blueberries
» 1 tablespoon ground flaxseeds
» 1 teaspoon of sunflower butter or 1 tablespoon of sunflower seeds
» ¼ lemon juice
» ½ cup cultured oat milk naturally flavored (blueberry) or plain kefir or a plain yogurt alternative (optional)
» 1 ½ cup of filtered water
» ½ cup ice cubes
» 1 teaspoon of honey or 1 date (optional)

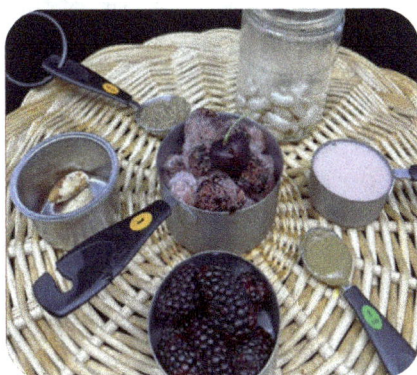

Pre preparation (you may skip this if you prefer to use drained and rinsed BPA-free canned cannellini beans)
1. Let this sleep overnight: one cup of filtered water and 1/4 cup beans.
2. The next day you will find that the beans have expanded to 1/2 cup. Pour away the water.
3. In a pot, add one cup of filtered water, the beans, a cinnamon stick and one clove.
4. Boil it on a medium temperature for 10 minutes.
5. After boiling, do not pour the remaining water away (you will probably be left with two spoons worth). Let it cool and then pour the entire contents into your blender.

Smoothie Preparation
1. Add all of the ingredients (including the clove and cinnamon) and blend until smooth. (If you used canned cannellini, add the cinnamon and clove directly to the blender.)
2. BON APPETITE!

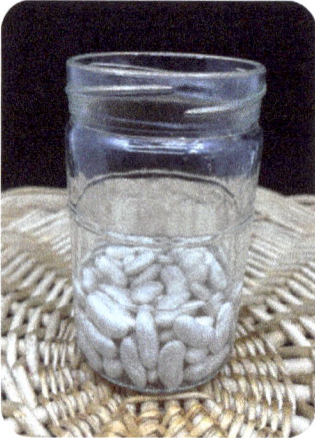

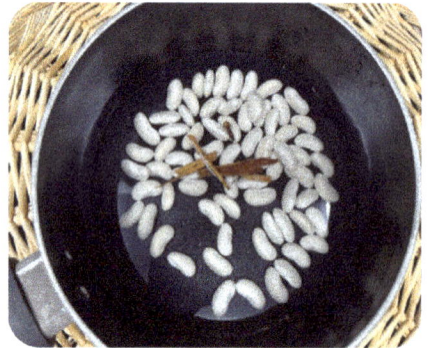

The Cherry on Top's Ingredients

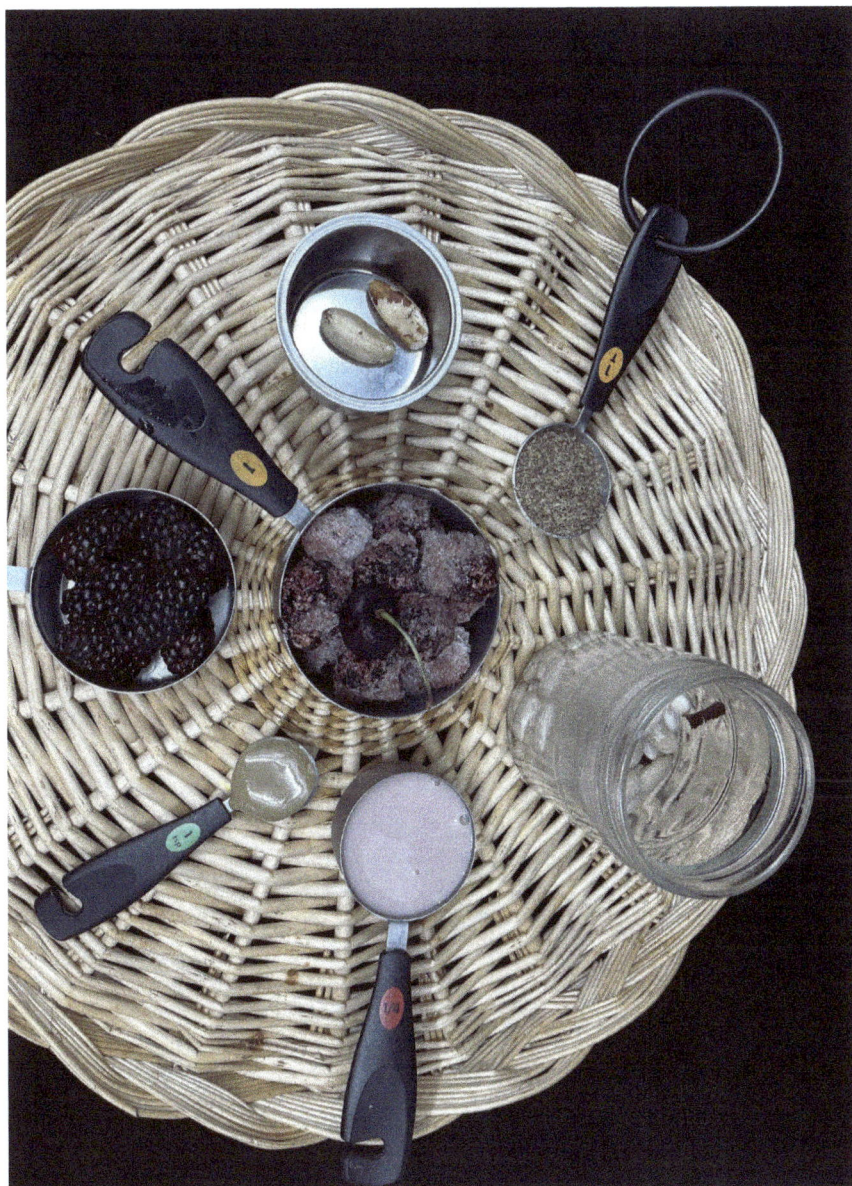

The Cherry on Top nutrition facts and benefits

NUTRITION FACTS (1 serving)

Calories: 129kcal
Carbohydrates: 22g
Protein: 6g
Fat: 6g
Saturated Fat: 0.5g
Cholesterol: 0mg
Sodium: 21mg
Potassium: 78 mg
Fiber: 7g
Sugar: 9g

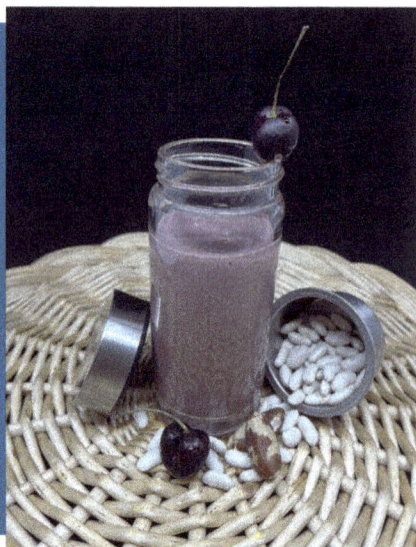

HEALTH BENEFITS: The antioxidant content of blueberries and blackberries work to support your health. The most significant part of blueberries' health advantages is played by anthocyanins. In addition, the volatiles from blueberries and blackberries may provide potential anti-cancer activity through apoptosis in lung cancer [51, 57]. Both ellagic acid and selenium, which are found in Brazil nuts, are good for your brain. Polyphenol ellagic acid is found in Brazil nuts. It offers both antioxidant and anti-inflammatory properties that may have protective and antidepressant effects on your brain [58]. Sunflower seeds include flavonoids as well as other plant components that decrease inflammation [59]. Cannellini beans provide nutrients such as iron, Folate, and vitamin B, all of which are essential for brain health. Research has shown that these nutrients foster the production of neurotransmitters, which are chemicals that help transmit signals in the brain [60].

Cherries could be Cherries could be an attractive candidate to formulate an agent for the prevention of oxidative which leads to stress-induced disorders such as intestinal inflammation disorders or an appropriated delivery system for neurodegenerative diseases an attractive candidate to formulate an agent for the prevention of oxidative. stress-induced disorders such as intestinal inflammation disorders or with an appropriated delivery system for neurodegenerative diseases [61]. Research on data suggests that cherries also offer an anti-fatiguing effect as well as the ability to improve sustained attention during times of high cognitive demand [62]. Kefir represents a potent antiviral agent against both viral hepatitis C and B, as well as having antimicrobial and wound healing potential [63]. It was found that exercising and consuming clove supplementation could improve memory by increasing the acetylcholine receptor (AChR) and decreasing pyrin domain containing 1 NLRP1 and dark cells [64].

Cinnamon increases sensitivity to the hormone insulin, having a potent anti-diabetic effect.

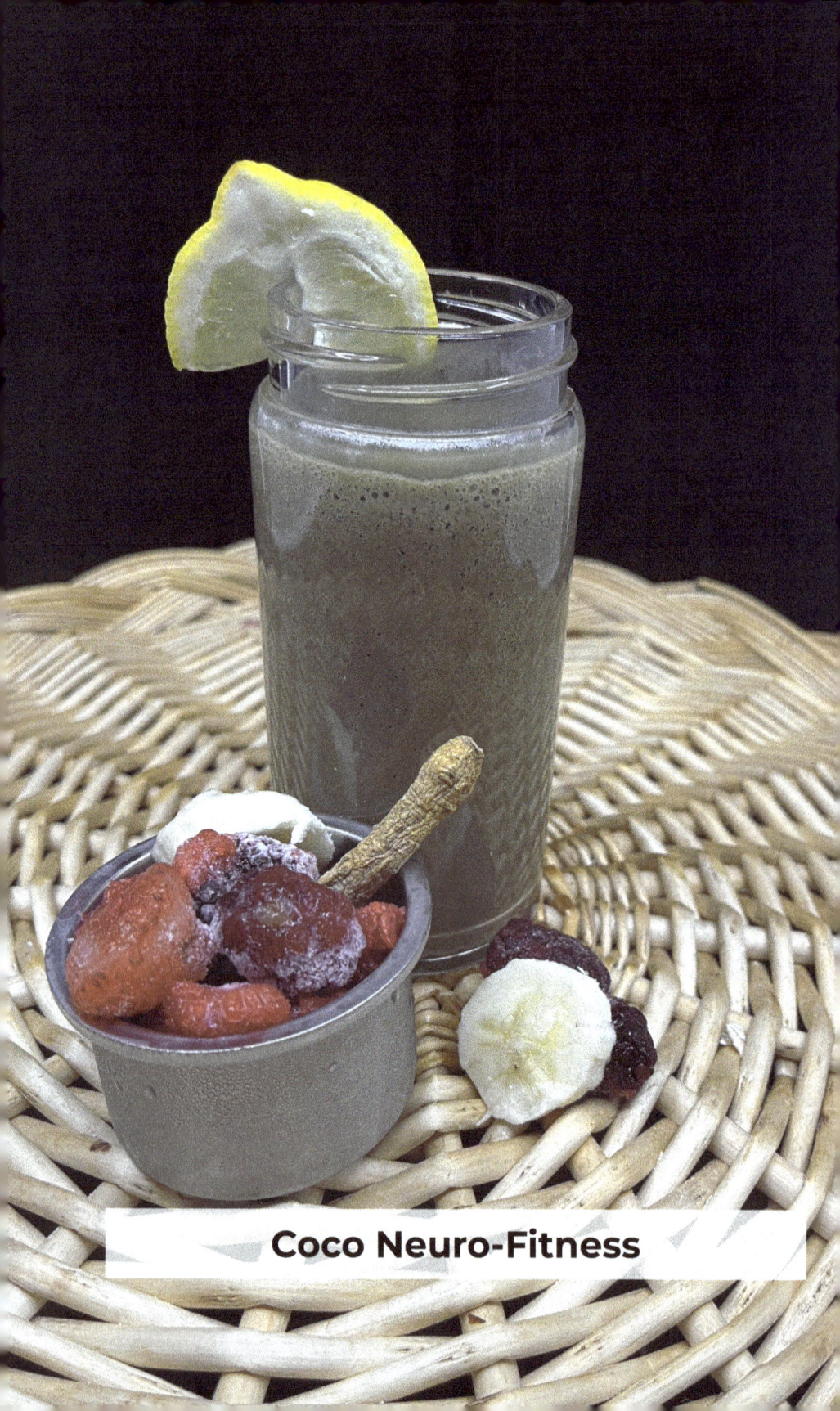

Coco Neuro-Fitness

ME3. Coco Neuro-Fitness

Experience the ultimate brain-boosting blend featuring kale, ginseng, protein powder, banana, and coconut oil. Berries enhance memory and mood, while ginseng may offer anti-Alzheimer's and neuroprotective benefits. Embrace the power of coconut oil to directly support cognitive function. Savor this nourishing elixir for a sharper mind and improved well-being.

INGREDIENTS

(Serves 1)

» 1/2 cup (plain or flavored) cultured low-fat milk (probiotic kefir) or cultured oat milk (contains probiotic)
» 1 cup fresh kale or spinach
» 1 cup of frozen berries
» 1 cup sliced ripe banana or half banana.
» 1 scoop of your favorite unflavored protein powder or collagen powder
» 1 tablespoon of ginseng (powder) or ginseng roots or Korean ginseng
» 1/4 tablespoon coconut oil (if you are not familiar with the flavor, begin with ¼ and then go to 1 tablespoon in the future)
» ¼ lemon juice
» 1/2 cup filtered water + 1/3 cup of ice cubes

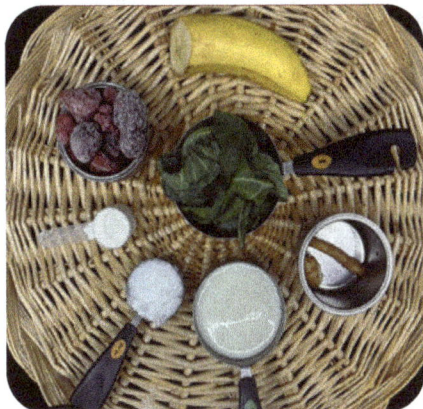

INSTRUCTIONS

1. Place all ingredients in a blender, cover and process until completely smooth.
2. BON APPETITE!

Coco Neuro-Fitness's Ingredients

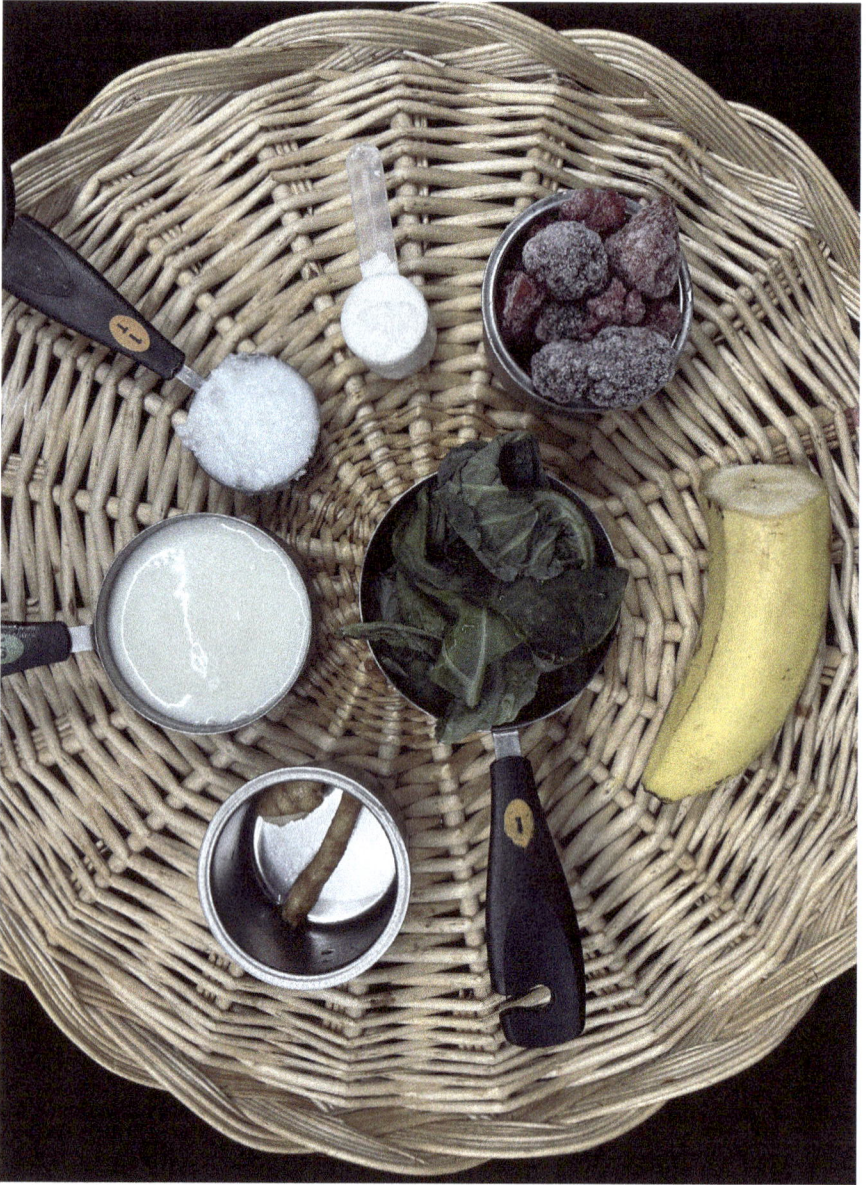

Coco Neuro-Fitness nutrition facts and benefits

NUTRITION FACTS (1 serving)

Calories: 215kcal
Carbohydrates: 29g
Protein: 10g
Fat: 8g
Saturated Fat: 1g
Cholesterol: 3mg
Sodium: 65mg
Potassium: 122mg
Fiber: 7g
Sugar: 17g

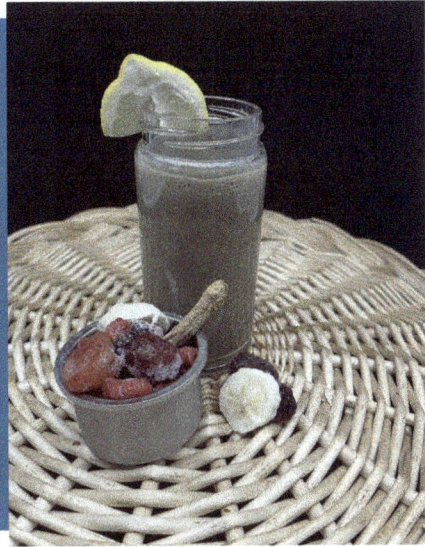

HEALTH BENEFITS: Zeaxanthin and lutein in spinach work to prevent macular degeneration and cataracts, which are major causes of blindness [24]. Kale is considered a superfood because its nutrients contain fiber, antioxidants, calcium, vitamins C and K, iron, as well as a wide range of other nutrients that can help prevent various health problems [65]. The flavonoids in berries have also been demonstrated to assist in improving balance, memory, and mood, according to a 2022 study published in scientific reports [66]. Researchers found that ginsenoside has potential anti-Alzheimer efficacy. Alzheimer's disease is a critical neurodegenerative disease that manifests as progressive intellectual decline and is pathologically characterized by a progressive loss of neurons in the brain [67]. Results have provided evidence that Korean ginseng and its constituents exert antidepressant effects [68]. Due to the composition and biological properties of coconut oil, there is still considerable debate regarding the potential benefits for the management of obesity, including the specific impact on body weight reduction in addition to there being promising evidence regarding the anti-inflammatory antioxidant, and neuroprotective properties of virgin coconut oil [69, 70]. Cultured plant based milk and kefir are rich in probiotic.

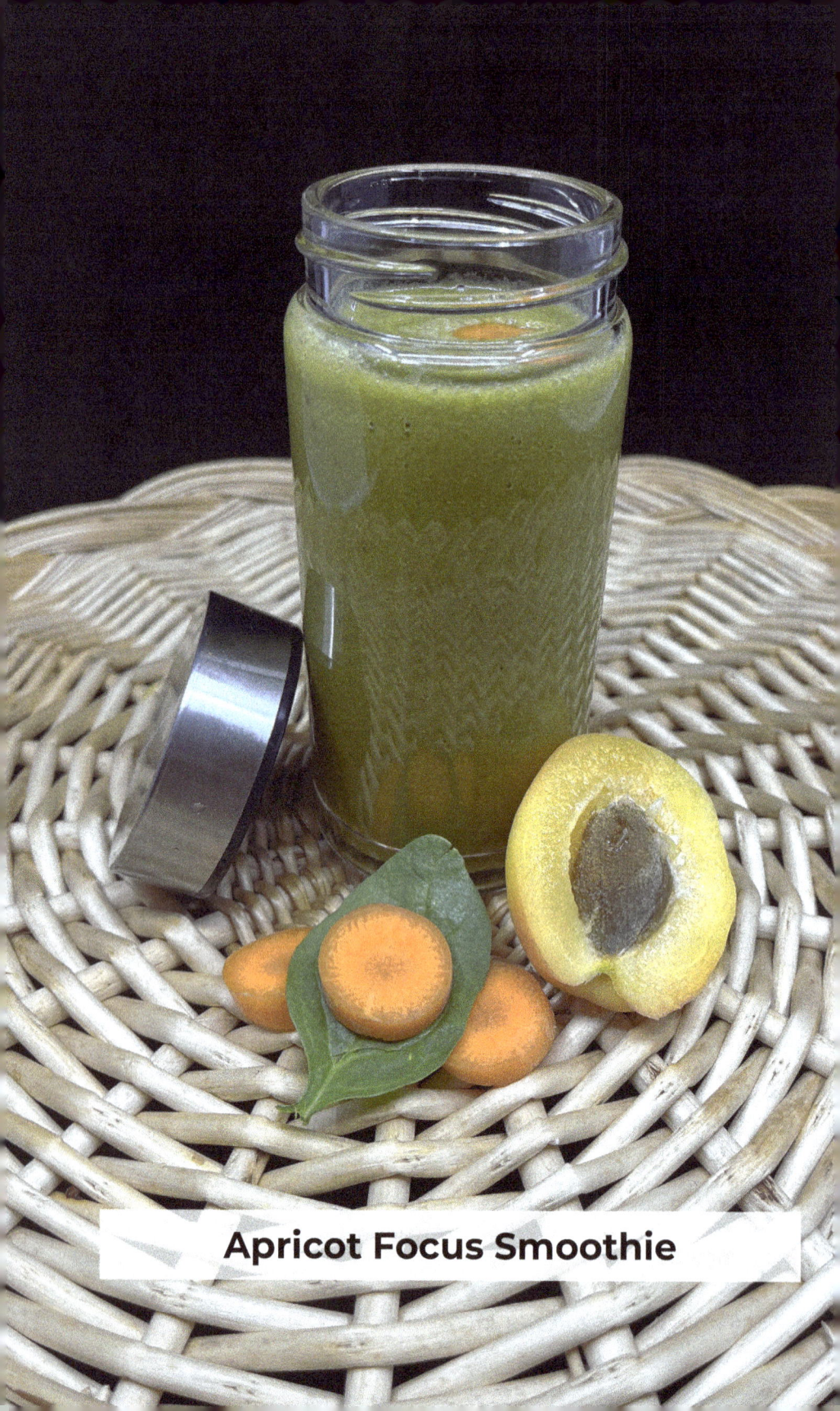

Apricot Focus Smoothie

ME4. Apricot Focus Smoothie

Embrace the potency of bacopa monnieri in this smoothie, delivering neuroprotective benefits against Parkinson's disease. Apricots, rich in lutein, work to prevent Alzheimer's disease, while carrot juice acts as a safeguard against neuronal damage. Sip your way to brain health with this nourishing blend of nature's wonders.

INGREDIENTS

(Serves 1)

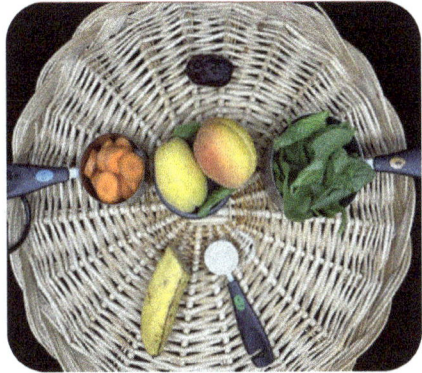

» 1 cup fresh spinach
» 2 white apricots with no seed or 1 cup of frozen white apricots
» ½ banana
» 1/3 cup raw carrots cut in pieces
» 1 tablespoon of bacopa monnieri
» 1 date (or one teaspoon of raw honey)
» ¼ teaspoon cinnamon
» 1 cup filtered water + 5 ice cubes

INSTRUCTIONS

1. Place all of the ingredients into your blender, cover, and then process until smooth.
2. BON APPETITE!

Apricot Focus Smoothie's Ingredients

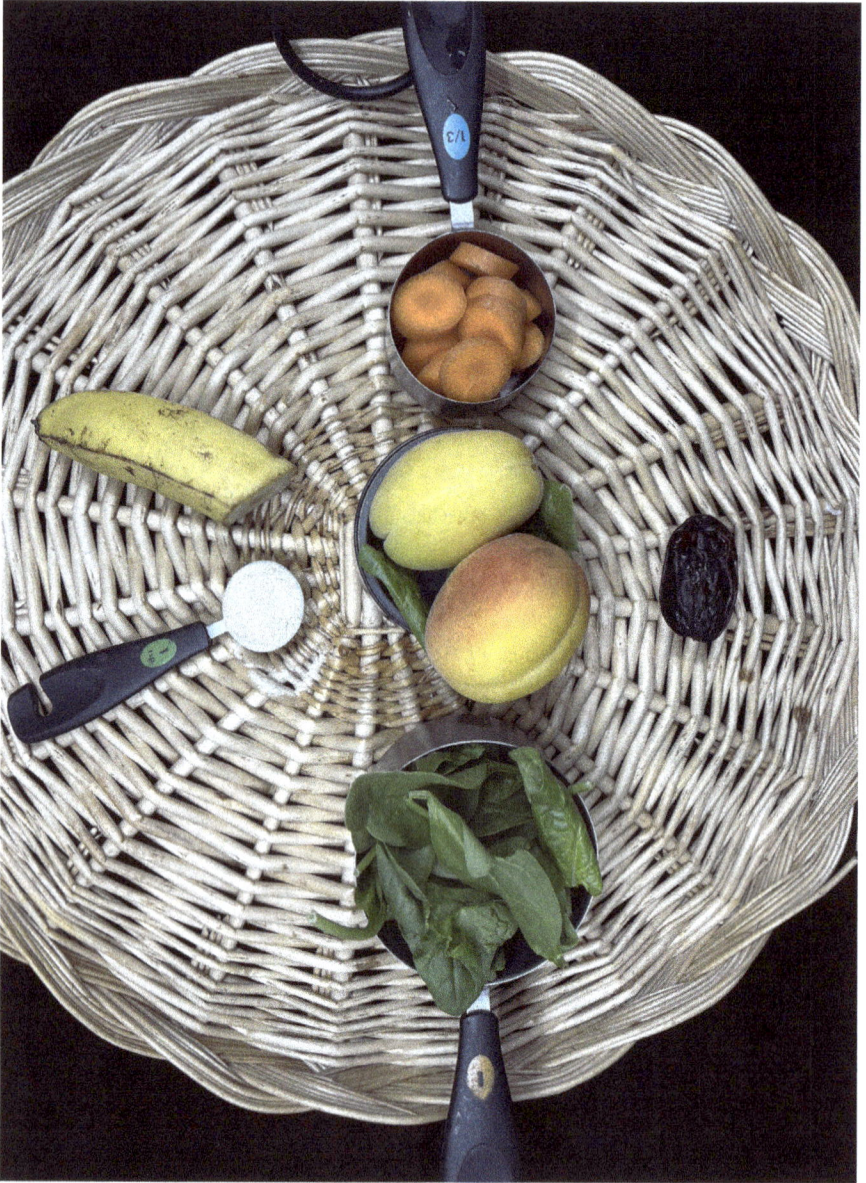

Apricot Focus Smoothie nutrition facts and benefits

NUTRITION FACTS (1 serving)

Calories: 215kcal
Carbohydrates: 29g
Protein: 10g
Fat: 8g
Saturated Fat: 1g
Cholesterol: 3mg
Sodium: 65mg
Potassium: 122mg
Fiber: 7g
Sugar: 17g

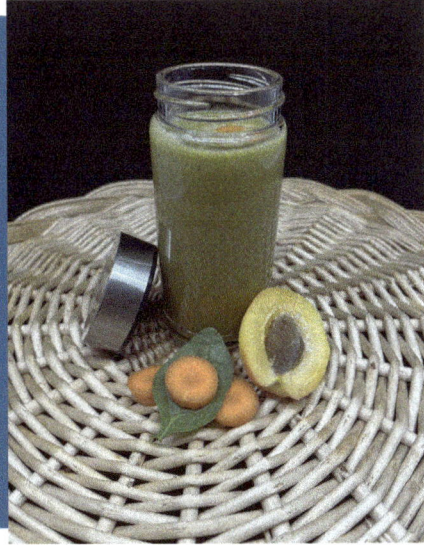

HEALTH BENEFITS: Zeaxanthin and lutein in spinach work to prevent macular degeneration and cataracts, which are major causes of blindness [22]. Brahmi from Bacopa monnieri has a potent antioxidant property and neuroprotective effects against Parkinson's disease that help reduce oxidative stress and neuroinflammation while enhancing dopamine levels [71]. Alzheimer's disease is the most common form of dementia and is characterized by the progressive accumulation of amyloid beta protein in areas of the brain, research findings suggest that lutein in fruits (such Apricot) may be useful as a preventive agent for amyloid-associated diseases [72]. The regulation of white apricot genes define a novel mechanism of action for thyroid hormone which can be important for its effects in developing the brain [73]. A study showed that the bioactive compounds in beetroot/carrot juice can modulate levels in neurons, and thus, potentially act as a neuroprotective factor against neuronal damage [74]. Dates are high in fiber, and the cinnamon reduces risk of the cholesterol.

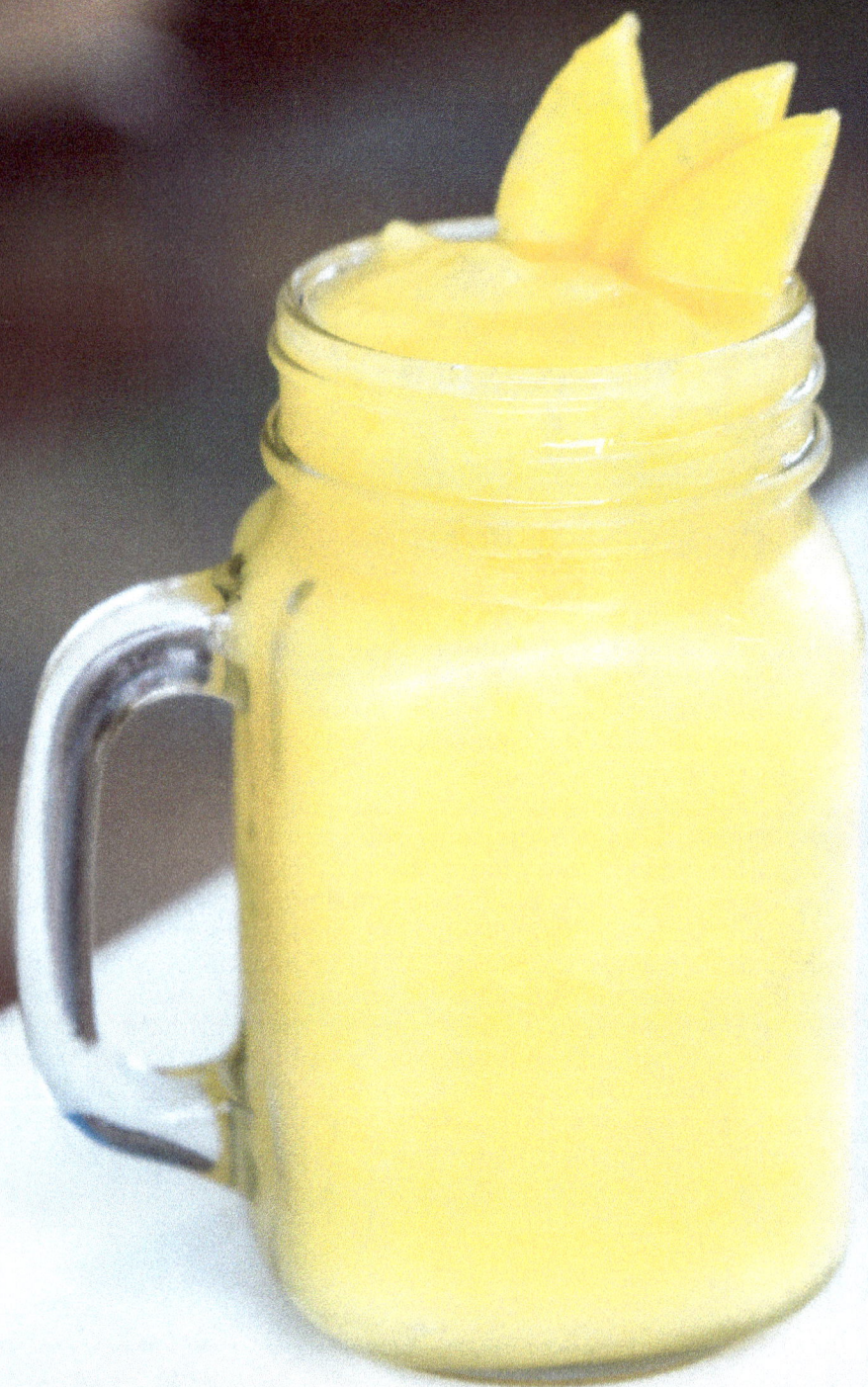
SMOOTH NEURODEGENERATIVE DISORDERS

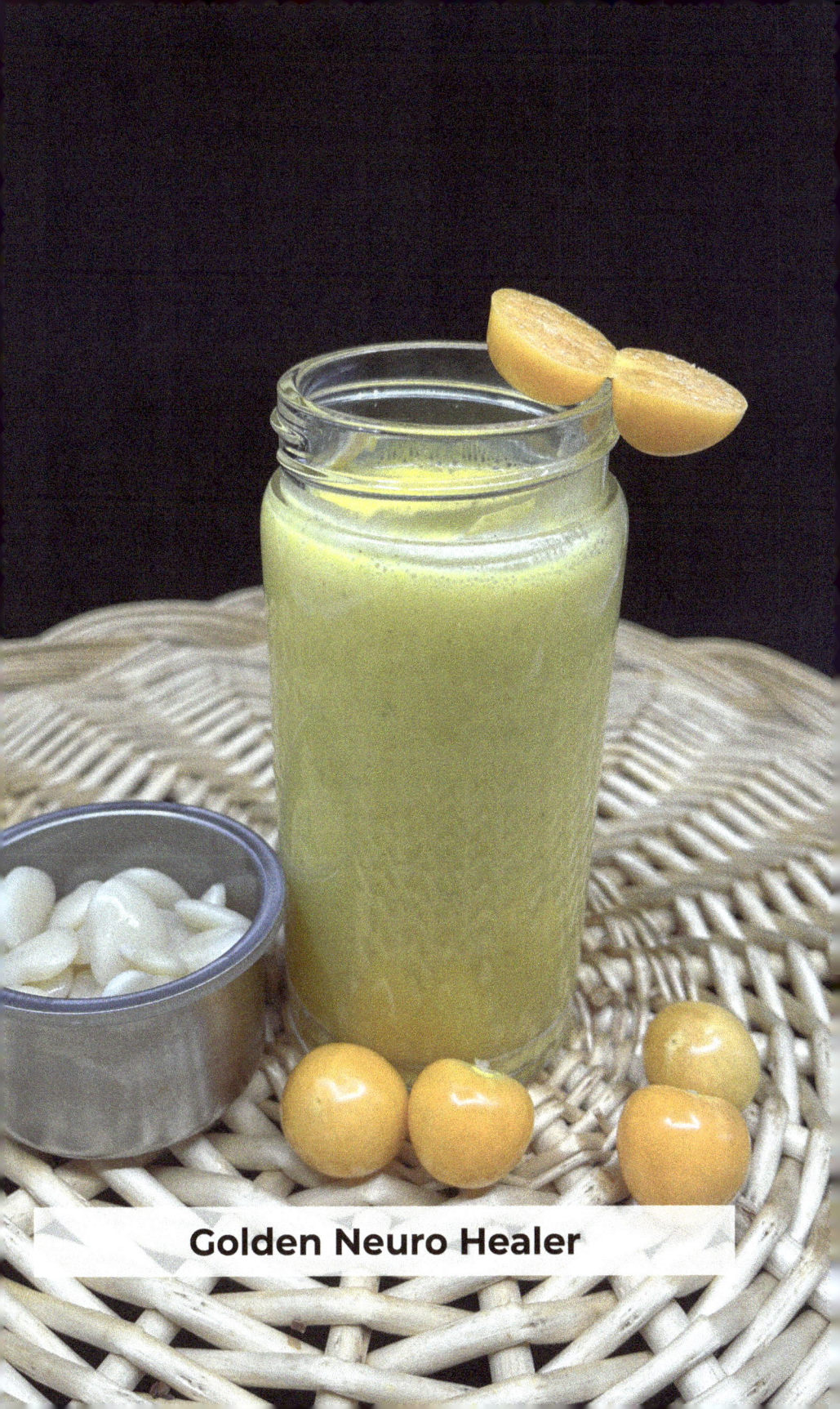

Golden Neuro Healer

ND1. Golden Neuro Healer

Experience the healing power of our Golden Neuro Healer smoothie! Fava beans and golden berries create an invincible shield against Parkinson's disease. Turmeric, Brazil nuts, and maca offer unparalleled brain support, while sunflower seeds and cinnamon reduce inflammation and manage diabetes. Feel the vitality coursing through your body with every sip of this magical blend.

INGREDIENTS

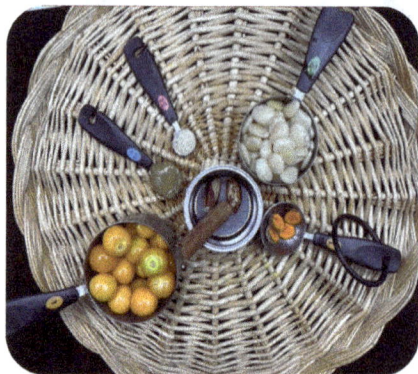

🔔 (Serves 1)

- » 2 raw Brazil nuts, chopped
- » ½ cup of cooked fava beans or kosher fava beans in a can
- » ¾ cup golden berries or blueberries
- » 1 tablespoon of maca
- » 1 tablespoon sunflower seeds or sunflower butter
- » 1 cinnamon stick or ¼ tablespoon cinnamon
- » 3 slides of turmeric
- » A pinch of black pepper
- » ½ cup cooked fava beans
- » 1 cup coconut water, ½ cup ice cubes

INSTRUCTIONS

The fava beans need to be cooked or use kosher fava beans from a can.

How to cook the fava beans

1. Let ½ cup beans sleep in one cup of filtered water for the night.
2. The next day you will see that the beans have grown to 1 cup. Pour the water and add a new (one) cup of filtered water. Then boil on a medium temperature for 10 minutes.

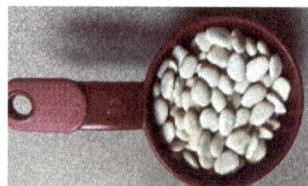

3. After boiling, pour away the water, and you will have one cup of cooked fava beans. You only need half of the cup for this smoothie recipe, so you can save the other half in the refrigerator to use within the next 72 hours.

Prepare smoothie!
1. Add all ingredients to the blender. Blend until smooth.
2. BON APPETITE!

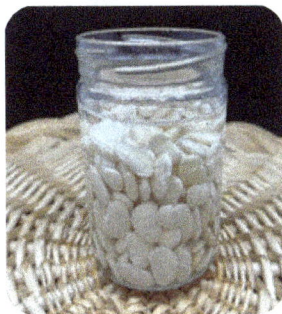

Golden Neuro Healer nutrition facts and benefits

**NUTRITION FACTS
(1 serving)**

Calories: 129kcal
Carbohydrates: 22g
Protein: 6g
Fat: 6g
Saturated Fat: 0.5g
Cholesterol: 0mg
Sodium: 21mg
Potassium 78 mg
Fiber: 7g
Sugar: 9g

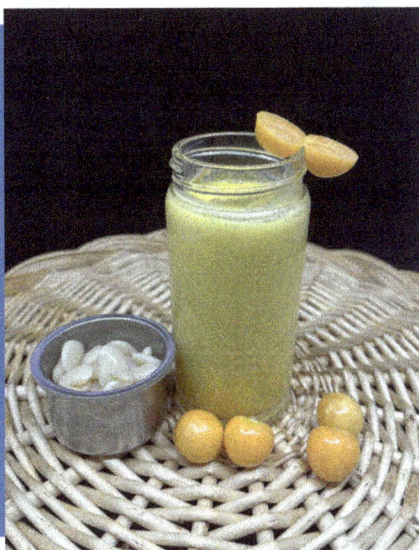

HEALTH BENEFITS: Golden berries possess a higher concentration of phytochemicals and antioxidants compared to other berries. These compounds play a crucial role in protecting the brain from oxidative stress and inflammation, which are implicated in age-related cognitive decline and neurodegenerative diseases (parkinsondisease.net). Moreover, golden berries (Physalis peruviana L.) have potential benefits relevant to risk reduction of cardiometabolic disease [15]. Collaborative findings indicate that blueberry supplementation in humans with mild cognitive impairment increased verbal memory performance [75]. Both ellagic acid and selenium, which are found in Brazil nuts, are good for your brain. Polyphenol ellagic acid is found in Brazil nuts. It has both antioxidant and anti-inflammatory properties that may have protective and antidepressant effects on your brain [58]. Sunflower seeds also include flavonoids and other plant components that decrease inflammation [59]. Fava beans get their own mention because they contain levodopa, the same chemical compound used in medications to treat Parkinson's. Beans in general provide nutrients such as iron, folate, and vitamin B, which are essential for brain health. Research has shown that these nutrients foster the production of neurotransmitters, which are chemicals that help transmit signals in the brain [60]. Maca plays a role in combating ameliorates oxidative stress, improving energy metabolism, and restoring mitochondrial respiration thereby preventing liver damage [76]. Cinnamon can be used as an anti-diabetic agent and an add-on treatment to control glycemic indices among patients with type 2 diabetes or polycystic ovary symptoms [77]. Research has revealed that maca is beneficial to social memory and that it restores social recognition impairments by augmenting the oxytocinergic neuronal pathways, which play an essential role in diverse social behaviors [78].

Golden Neuro Healer's Ingredients

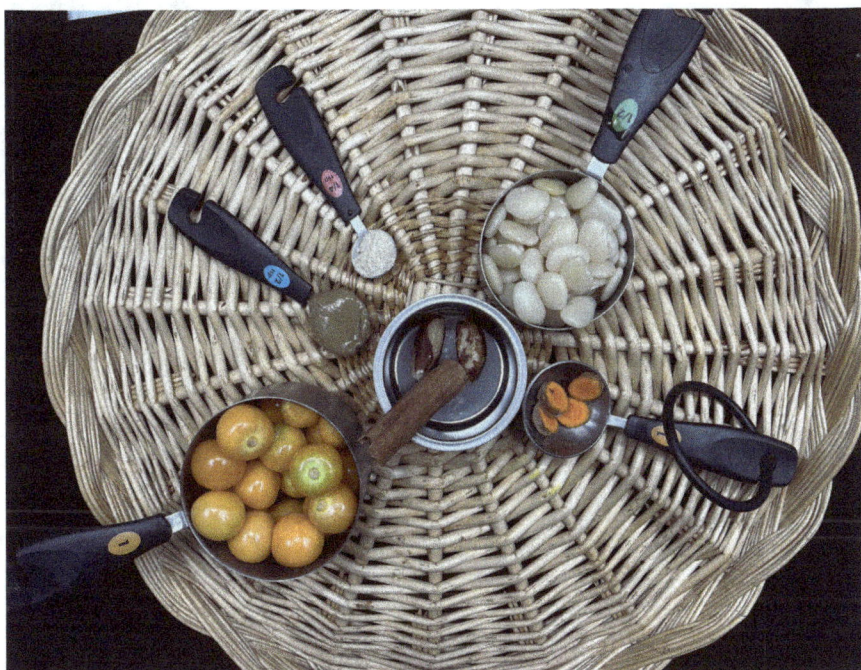

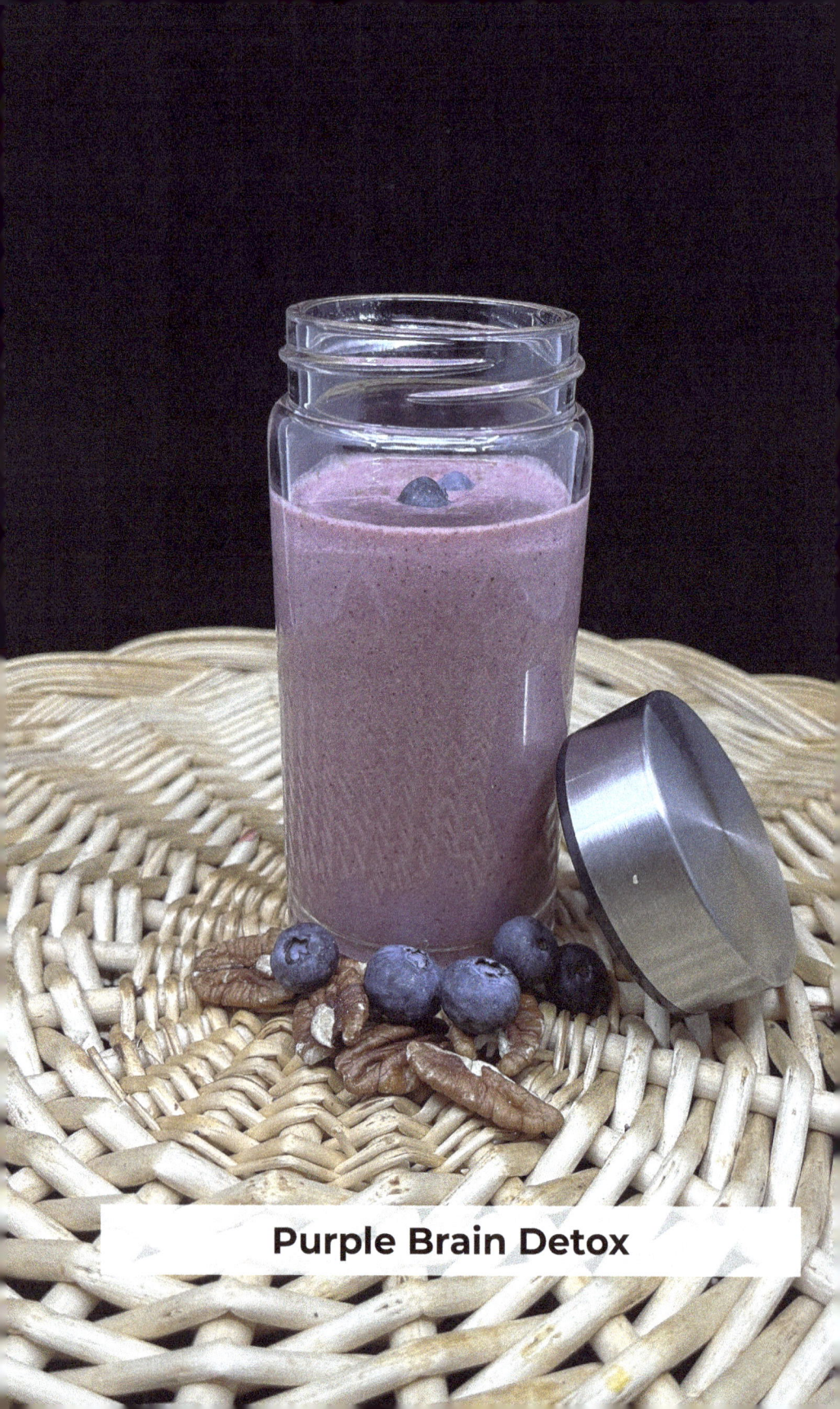
Purple Brain Detox

ND2. Purple Brain Detox

Experience the rejuvenating power of our Purple Brain Detox smoothie! Blueberries reverse age-related cognitive deficits, while strawberries unleash antioxidants. Turmeric disrupts the toxic loop of Parkinson's disease. Meanwhile, coconut milk and water suppress inflammation, and pecans prevent obesity. Embrace cognitive brilliance and defy aging with every sip of this extraordinary blend.

INGREDIENTS

(Serves 1)

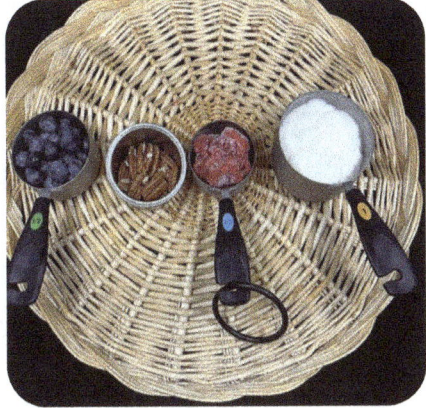

- » 1/3 cup strawberries (frozen or not)
- » ½ cup blueberries (frozen or not)
- » 10 half pecans
- » 2 slides of turmeric or 1 teaspoon of turmeric powder
- » A pinch of black pepper
- » ½ cup coconut water or filtered water
- » ½ cup plain yogurt or coconut yogurt alternative
- » Optional: 1 teaspoon of raw honey or manuka honey topped over the smoothie

INSTRUCTIONS

1. Place all the ingredients in a blender. Add 1/3 cup of ice (5 ice cubes) if desired.
2. Blend it until smooth.
3. Serve with 1 teaspoon of honey topped over the smoothie (this step is optional)
4. BON APPETITE!

Purple Brain Detox's Ingredients

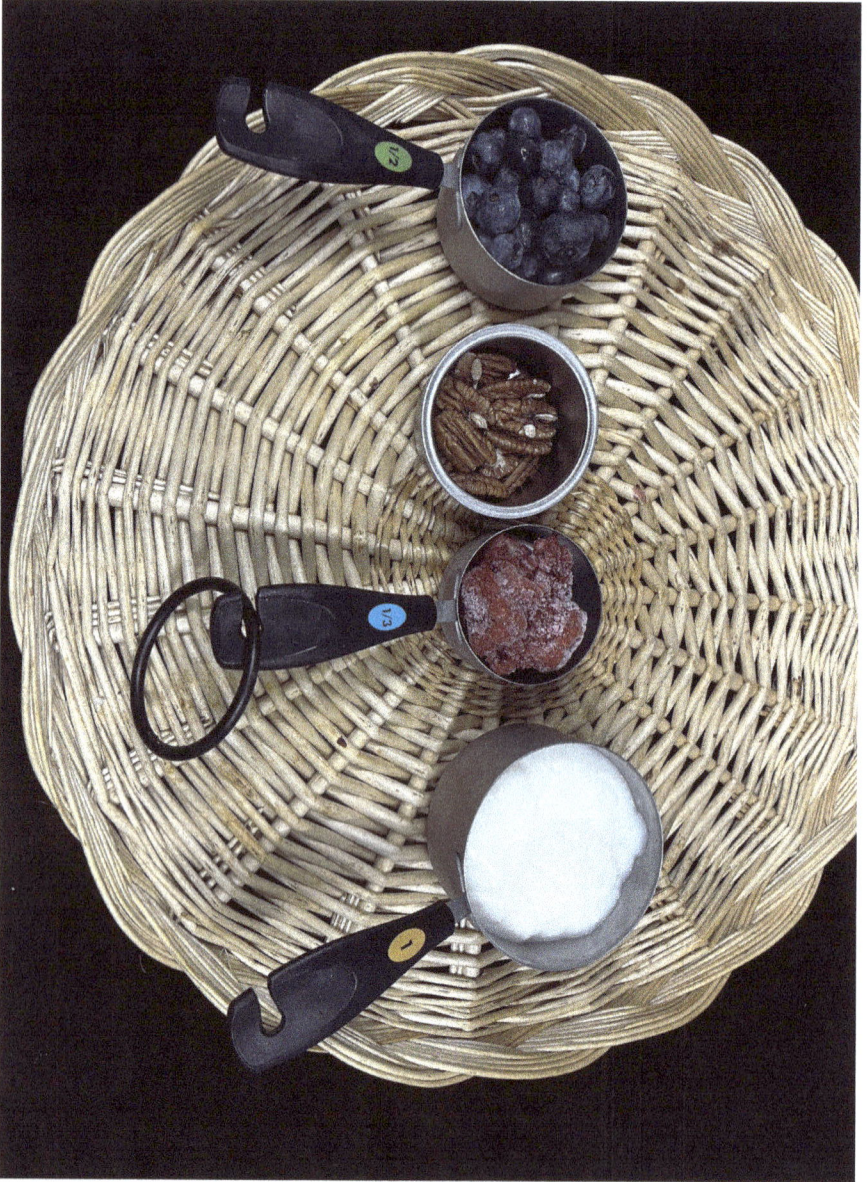

Purple Brain Detox nutrition facts and benefits

NUTRITION FACTS (1 serving)

Calories: 216.5 kcal
Carbohydrates: 38.9g
Protein: 6.5g
Fat: 4.6g
Saturated Fat: 2.8g
Cholesterol: 16mg
Sodium: 261.5mg
Potassium: 843mg
Fiber: 5.2g

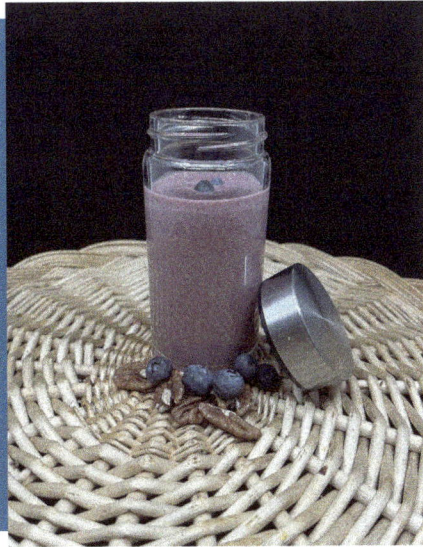

HEALTH BENEFITS: The antioxidant content of blueberries is thought to be among the highest of all commonly consumed fruits and vegetables. The most significant part of blueberries' health advantages is that they have a greater dietary intake and higher blood levels of antioxidants. The consumption of blueberries may reverse some age-related deficits in cognition, as well as preserve function among those with intact cognitive ability [79]. It was found that pecans prevented obesity, liver steatosis and diabetes by reducing dysbiosis, inflammation, and increasing mitochondrial content and energy expenditure [80]. Turmeric was found to be an attractive candidate to support the increase of reactive oxygen species, while iron may be important for disrupting the toxic loop that can cause Parkinson's disease [81]. Coconut milk and coconut water could ameliorate intestinal dysmotility associated with heat stress via oxidative stress reduction and the suppression of inflammatory responses [79, 82]. Strawberries contain high levels of antioxidants, which have been correlated with a decreased risk of chronic disease [83].

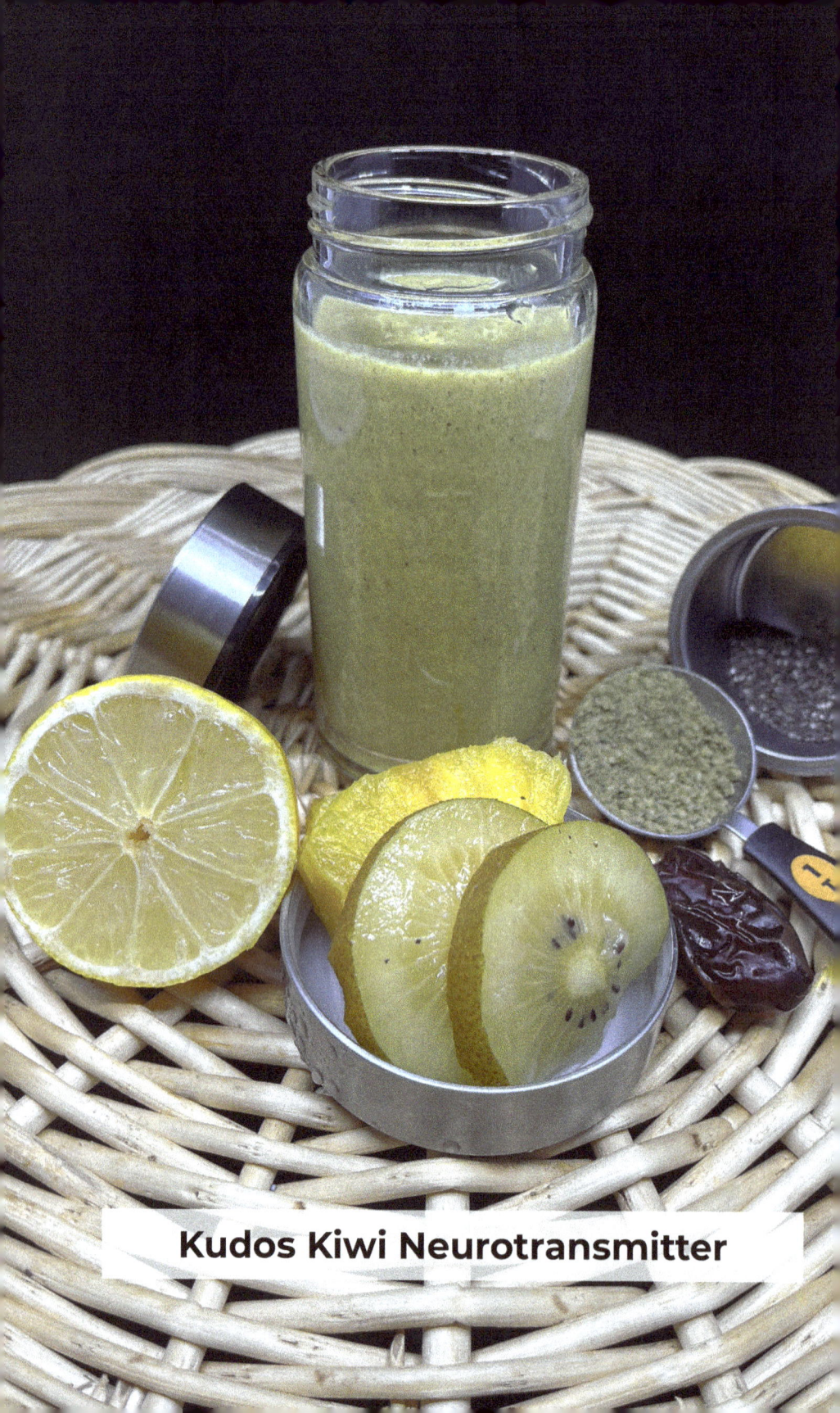

Kudos Kiwi Neurotransmitter

ND3. Kudos Kiwi Neurotransmitter

Embrace a burst of neurotransmitter support with our Kudos Kiwi Neurotransmitter smoothie! Kiwis, dates, and turmeric unite to combat neurodegenerative disorders. Chia, pineapple, and hemp seeds prevent inflammation and promote optimal brain health. Celebrate life and vitality with every sip of this invigorating blend!

INGREDIENTS

🍽 (Serves 2)

» 1 medium size kiwi
» 1 cup of pineapple chucks or 2 slices of pineapple
» ½ lemon squeezed
» ½ cup plain cultured low-fat milk probiotic (kefir) or cultured plant-based milk (contains probiotic)
» 1 date
» 1 tablespoon chia
» 1 tablespoon hemp hearts
» A pinch of cinnamon
» 3 slides of turmeric
» Pinch of black pepper
» 1 cup of water

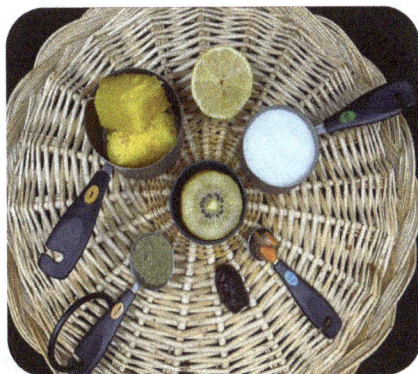

INSTRUCTIONS

1. Add kiwi, pineapple, turmeric, water, and yogurt or kefir in a blender. Blend until smooth.
2. Then add lemon, chia, hemp hearts, cinnamon, and black pepper. Blend again.
3. Finally, add 5 ice cubes and blend again if consistency is very thick.
4. BON APPETITE!

Kudos Kiwi Neurotransmitter's Ingredients

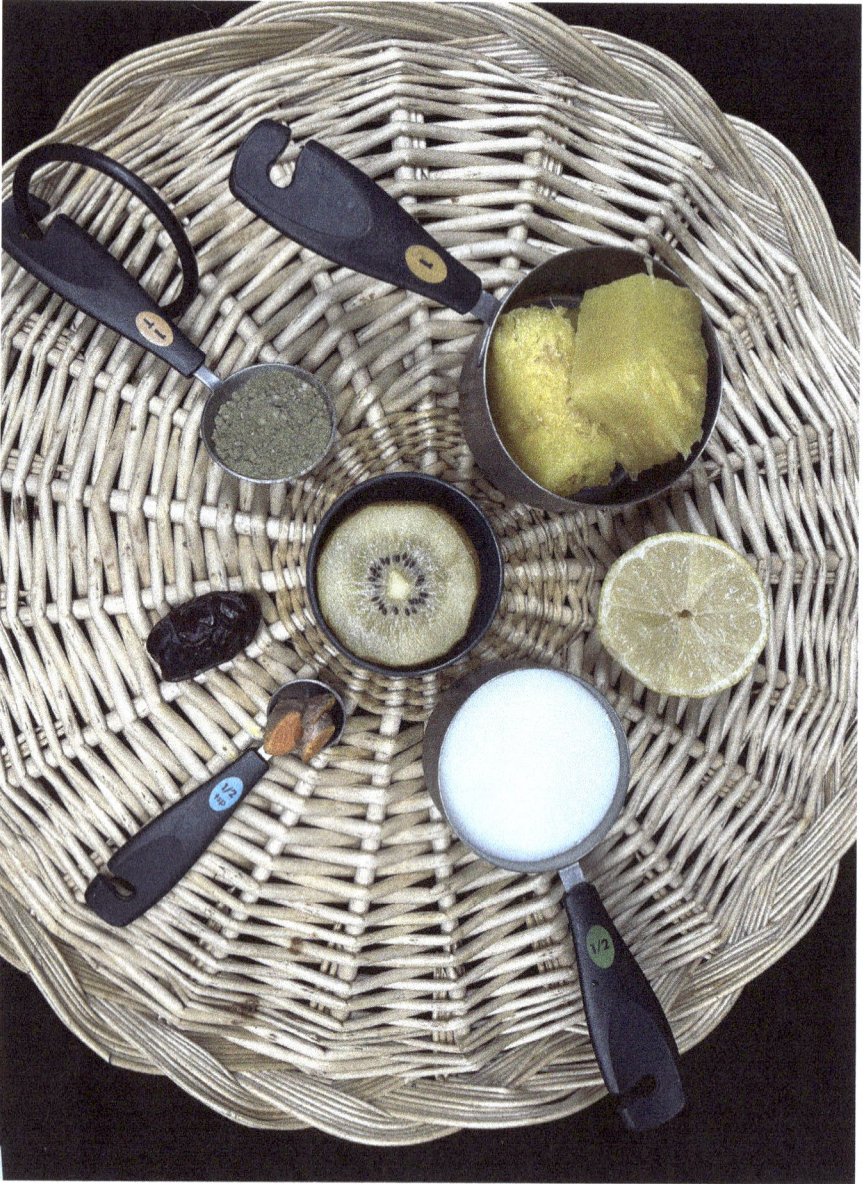

Kudos Kiwi Neurotransmitter nutrition facts and benefits

NUTRITION FACTS (1 serving)

Calories: 207.5kcal
Carbohydrates: 39.34g
Protein: 5.9g
Fat: 4.5g
Saturated Fat: 2.5g
Cholesterol: 16mg
Sodium: 60.5mg
Potassium: 649 mg
Fiber: 4.7g

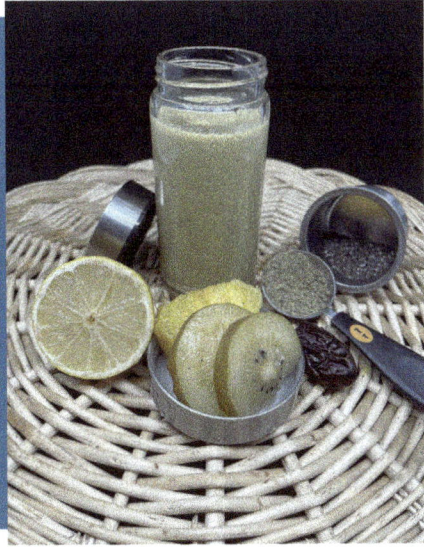

HEALTH BENEFITS: Carotenoids, which are found in kiwis, have positive effects on health. These substances comprise of lutein, zeaxanthin, and carotene beta. According to studies, eating foods high in carotenoids may help prevent some illnesses, such as cardiovascular diseases and neurogenerative disorders [51]. Kiwis contain extraordinarily high levels of vitamin C, which acts as a potent antioxidant in the body to shield cells from oxidative damage. Your body needs it to manufacture collagen and neurotransmitters [84]. It was found that intra-amniotic administration of the hydrolyzed chia protein or a probiotic, promoted positive changes in terms of intestinal inflammation, and morphology, thus improving intestinal health [85]. Turmeric offers the great potential of curcumin microemulsion for targeting the brain when it comes to the effective treatment of neurological ailments [86]. Studies of dates demonstrated an efficient method for preventing traumatic brain deterioration [87]. Foods containing hemp seeds might represent a source of healthy fats that are not likely to exacerbate the metabolic consequences of obesogenic diets while producing intestinal permeability protective effects as well as some anti-inflammatory actions [88]. Dates have strong antioxidants that can help premature aging.

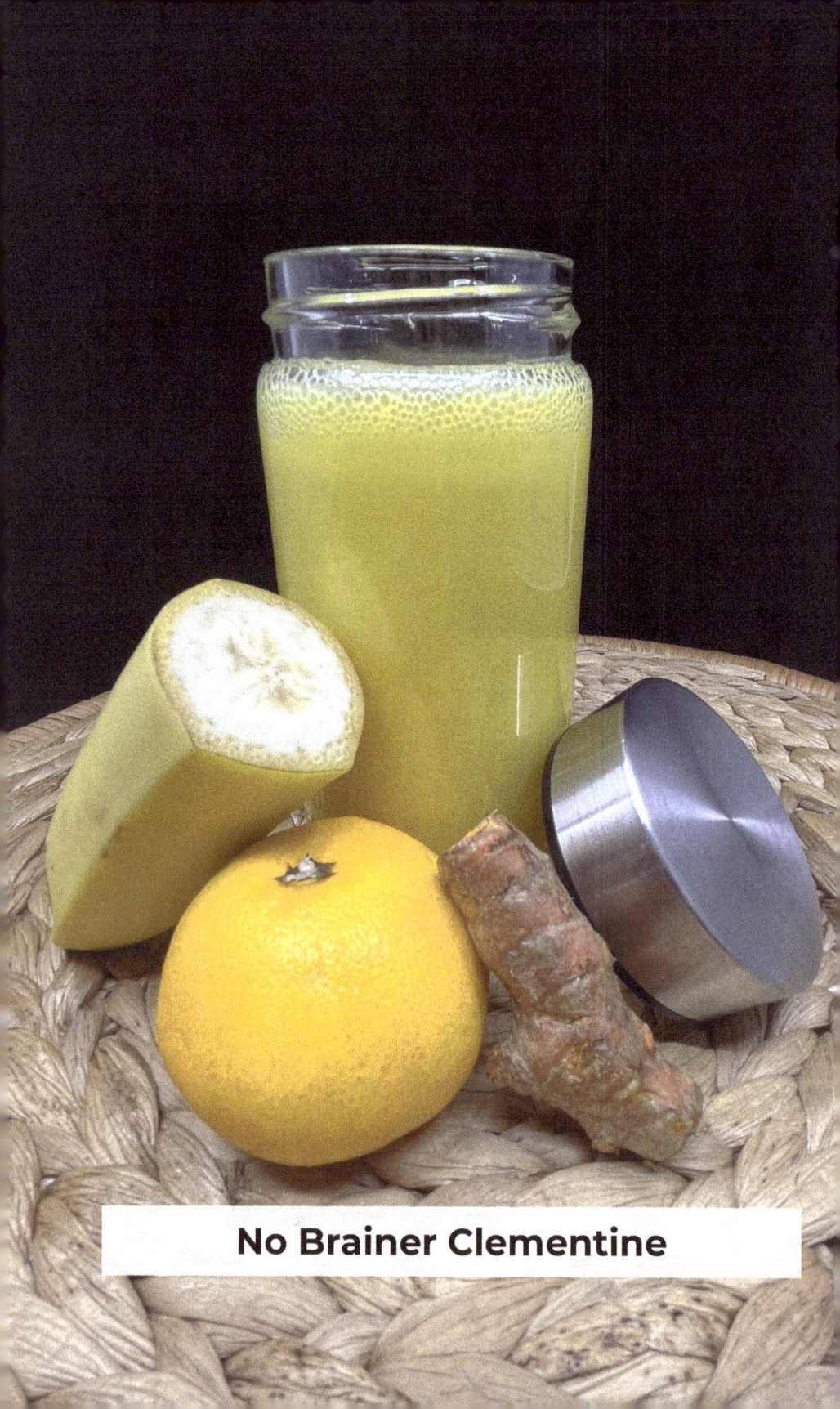
No Brainer Clementine

ND4. No Brainer Clementine

Experience the magic of our No Brainer Clementine smoothie! Clementine, banana, turmeric, and coconut milk unite to combat brain cell-damaging diseases like Parkinson's, Alzheimer's, and dementia. Embrace the simplicity and power of these ingredients as they invigorate your mind and protect your precious memories. A revitalizing treat for your brain awaits!

INGREDIENTS

(Serves 1)

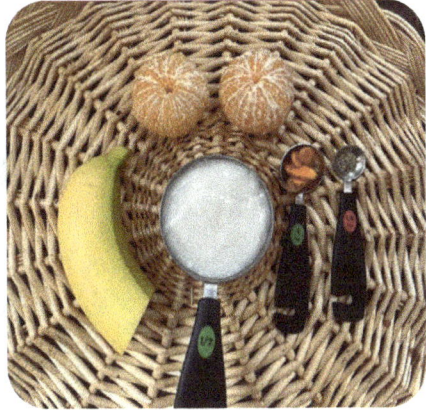

» 2 clementines
» ½ small banana
» ½ cup yogurt alternative (from coconut milk or almond milk)
» 1 teaspoon turmeric
» 1/8 teaspoon black pepper
» 1 teaspoon of raw honey
» 1/8 teaspoon of sea salt
» ½ cup of ice
» Suggested: add 1 teaspoon of maca

INSTRUCTIONS

1. Peel the clementines and banana, then cut the fruit into small chunks or slices.
2. Add the clementine slices, banana chunks, plain yogurt and turmeric in a blender and blend until smooth.
3. Add black pepper, sea salt and honey for taste.

No Brainer Clementine's Ingredients

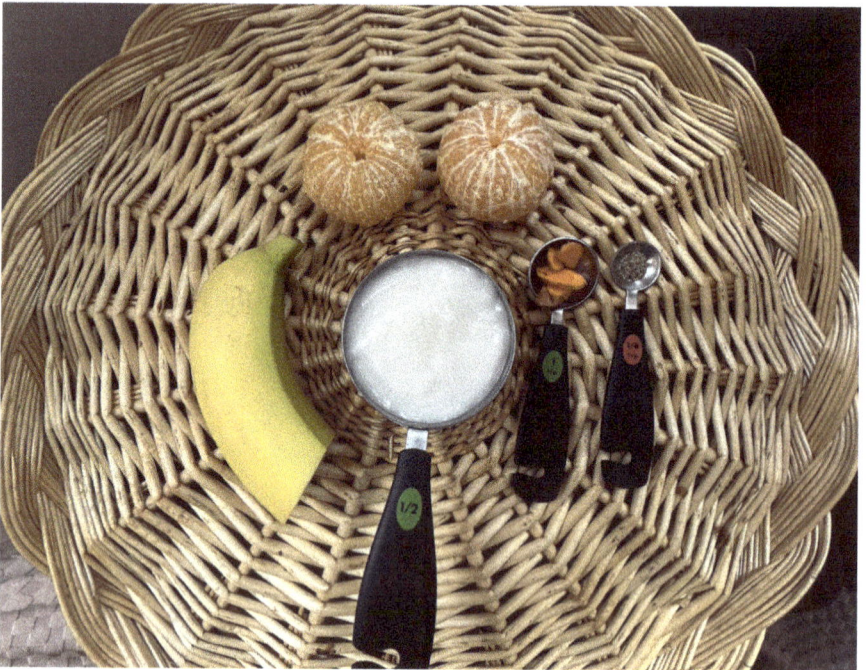

No Brainer Clementine nutrition facts and benefits

**NUTRITION FACTS
(1 serving)**

Calories: 190.5kcal
Carbohydrates: 34.4g
Protein: 5.9g
Fat: 4.27g
Saturated Fat: 2.5g
Cholesterol: 16mg
Sodium: 58.5mg
Potassium: 633mg
Fiber: 3.8g

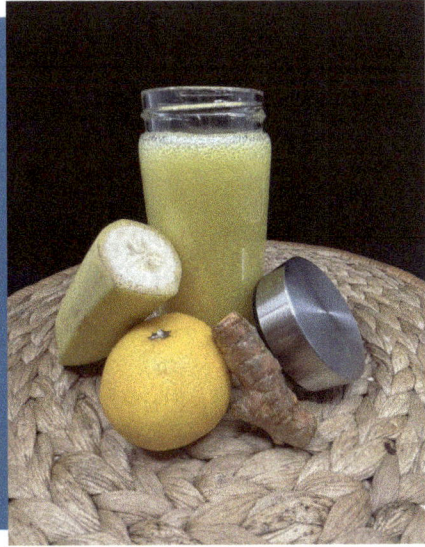

HEALTH BENEFITS: Clementines contain flavonoids that aid in the fight against diseases that harm brain cells, such as Parkinson's, Alzheimer's, and dementia [89].

Citrus fruit flavonoids offer anti-inflammatory properties and are thought to help fend off the series of events that lead to the degeneration of the nervous system. It has been demonstrated in mice and test-tube research that particular forms of flavonoids, such as hesperidin and apigenin, protect brain cells and enhance brain function [90]. Turmeric with curcumin microemulsion, has great potential for brain targeting in the effective treatment of neurological ailments [86]. Sea salt has been found to fight hypertension, kidney damage and psoriasis [91, 92]. Raw honey delivers anti-inflammatory properties [93].

Plant based yogurt is great for lactose intolerance, and they are packed with probiotics and support digestive system.

SMOOTHIES TO REDUCE ANXIETY AND DEPRESSION

Depression is categorized as being one of the most prevalent psychological disorders, and in recent times, its occurrence has risen, posing an escalating threat to public health. This analysis primarily aims to elucidate the significance and role of specific nutrients in one's diet and the consequences of nutrient insufficiencies on the likelihood of experiencing depression. Inadequate levels of vital nutrients, including protein, B vitamins, vitamin D, magnesium, zinc, selenium, iron, calcium, and omega-3 fatty acids, exert a notable influence on the functioning of the brain and nervous system, thereby impacting the manifestation of depressive symptoms. Nonetheless, it is crucial to acknowledge that diet alone does not solely determine the risk of developing or aiding in the treatment of depression. Various other factors, such as physical activity, sleep patterns, stress management, and social support, also hold substantial importance in maintaining mental well-being [94, 95]. There is a strong link between stress-induced depression and anxiety (DA) as well as gastrointestinal inflammation and dysbiosis. These conditions can lead to a reduction in brain-derived neurotrophic factor (BDNF) levels. Based on these discoveries, it has been suggested that a combination of probiotics that promote BDNF expression and L-theanine, known for its anti-inflammatory properties, may have an additive or synergistic effect in alleviating stress-induced depression and anxiety (DA) as well as gut dysbiosis. This combination can potentially regulate inflammation mediated by the gut microbiota and enhance BDNF expression, thus offering potential benefits for individuals suffering from DA [95].

Cognitive decline, anxiety, and depression have a substantial impact on overall human well-being and can lead to a decrease in the quality of life. The consumption of fruits, including 100% juice, has been linked to positive effects on various health outcomes [96].

SMOOTHIES TO REDUCE ANXIETY AND DEPRESSION

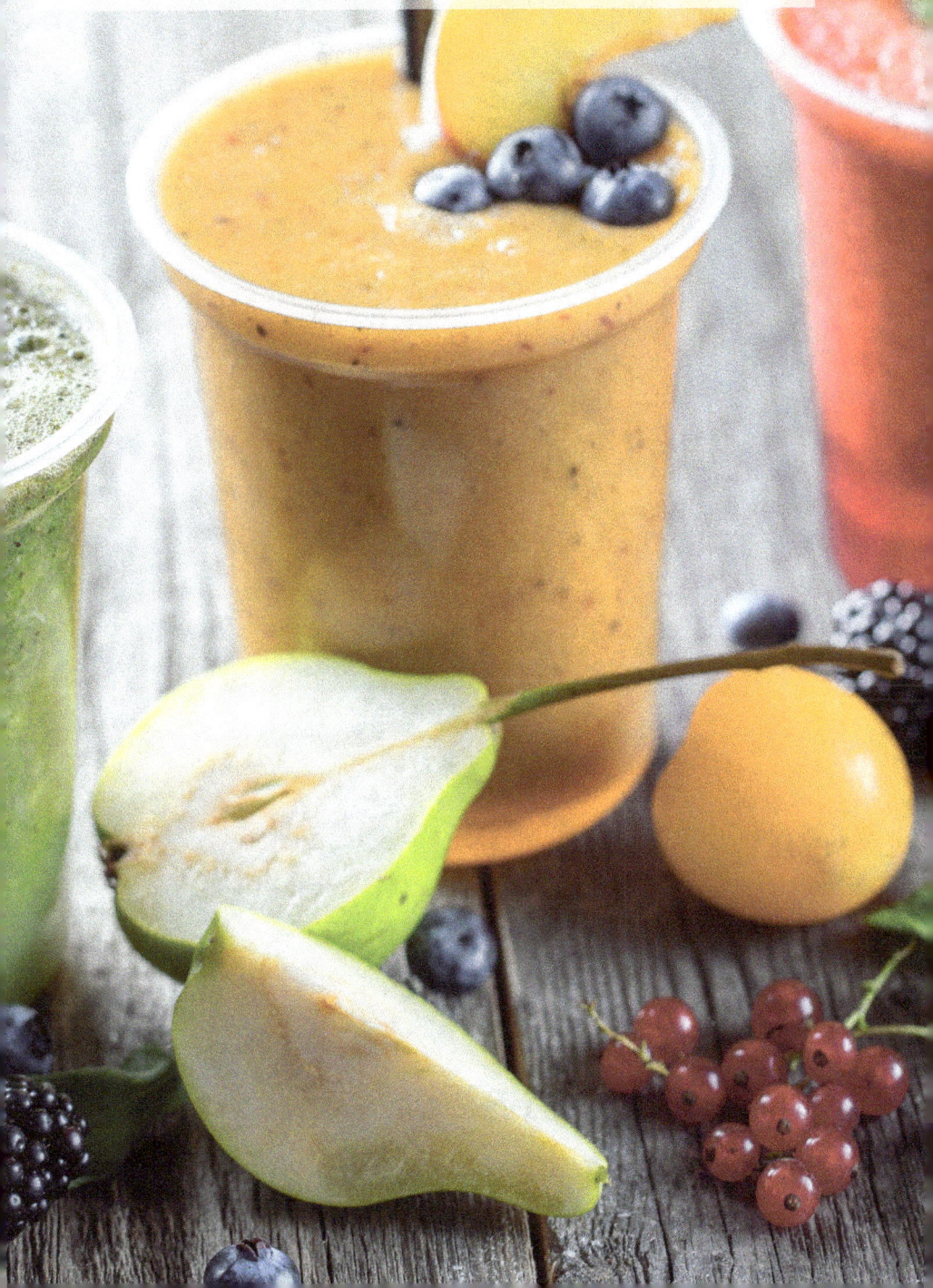

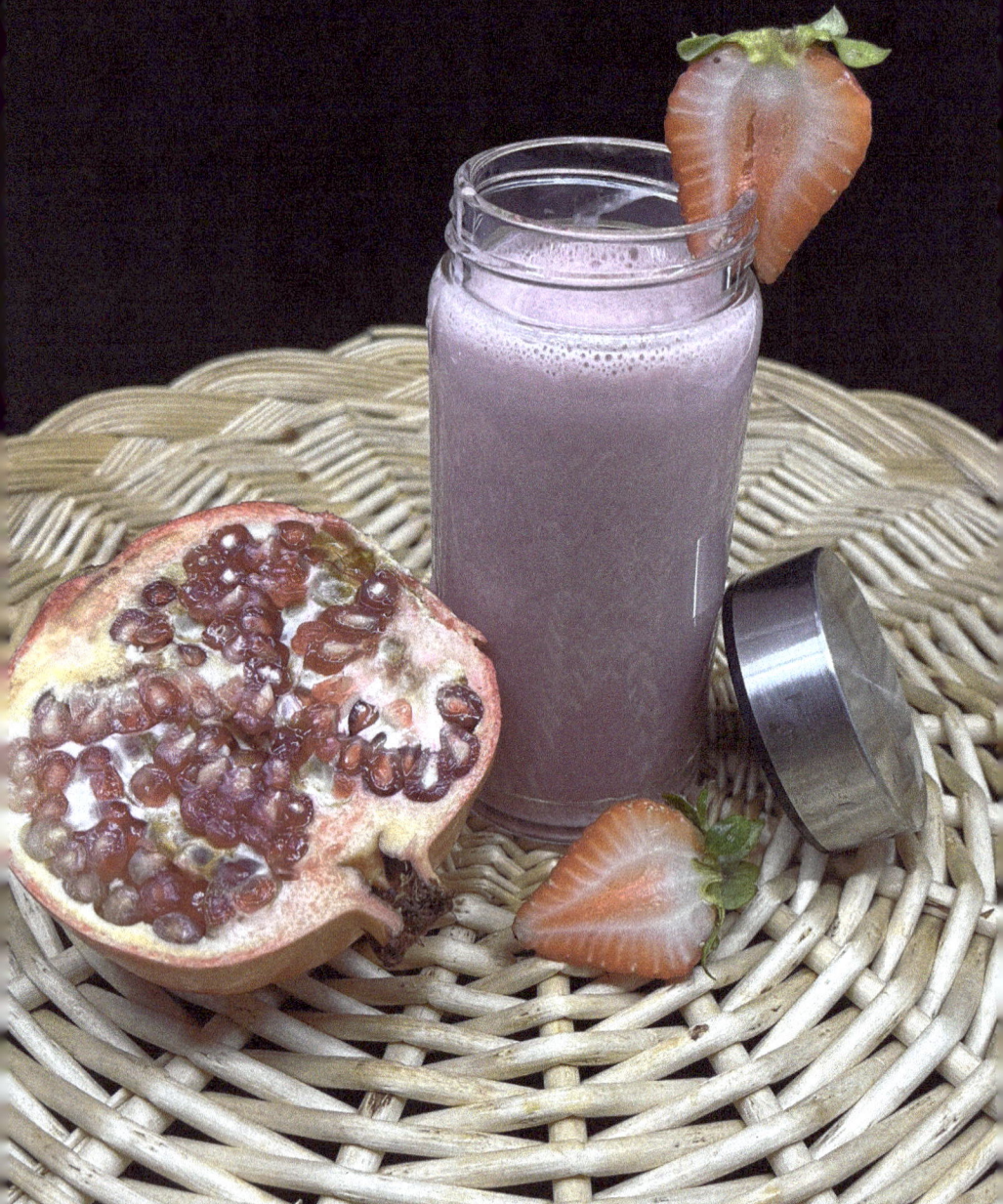

Relax, Psych Biotic Pomegranate!

MH1. Relax, Psych Biotic Pomegranate!

Delight in the ultimate relaxation with this sensational smoothie! Cultured oat milk and rolled oats team up for a neuroprotective psych-biotic effect, leaving you feeling invigorated. Experience the magic of anxiety-moderating pomegranate, while Brazil nuts and ginseng deliver a powerhouse of neuroprotective properties that will leave you beaming with joy. Embrace the blissful benefits of this incredible blend!

INGREDIENTS

(Serves 1)

» 1 cup of pomegranate
» ½ cup of strawberries
» 1/2 cup (plain or flavored) cultured low-fat milk (probiotic kefir) or cultured oat milk (contains probiotic)
» ¼ cup rolled oats (prebiotic)
» 2 Brazil nuts
» 1 teaspoon of ginseng
» 1/2 teaspoon of manuka honey
» 1/2 cup of water (if required to thin consistency)
» 5 ice cubes

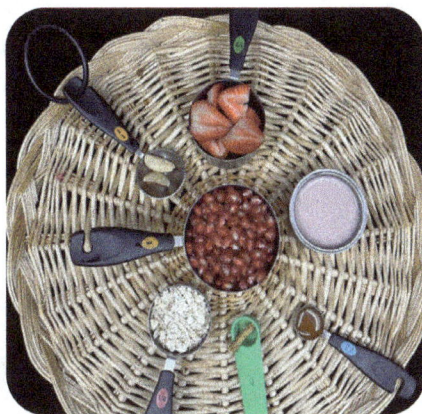

INSTRUCTIONS

1. Wash and cut down the strawberries into small chunks.
2. Put the cultured low-fat milk and strawberries into the blender and blend until smooth.
3. Add ½ cup water if consistency is thick.
4. Top the smoothie with 2-3 chopped strawberries and ½ teaspoon of honey (this step is optional).

Relax, Psych Biotic Pomegranate's Ingredients

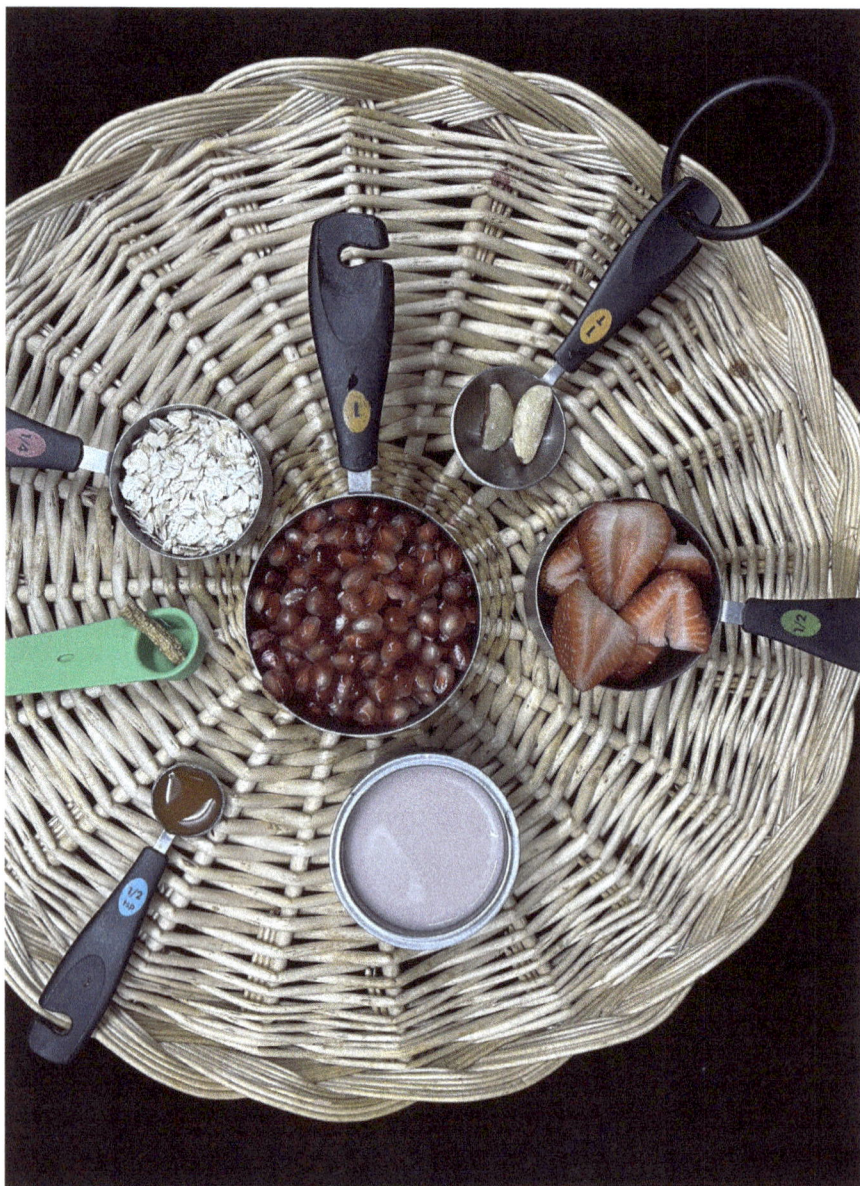

Relax, Psych Biotic Pomegranate! Nutrition facts and benefits

NUTRITION FACTS (1 serving)

Calories: 203kcals
Carbohydrates: 27.5g
Protein: 14g
Fat: 4.2g
Saturated Fat: 2.4g
Cholesterol: 14mg
Sodium: 173mg
Potassium: 725mg
Fiber: 2.3g

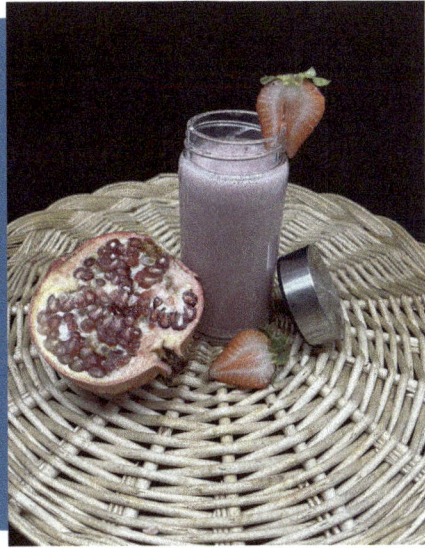

HEALTH BENEFITS: Strawberries contain a good amount of potassium, folate (vitamin B9), and manganese. Moreover, they are a great source of vitamin C and manganese. The high antioxidant and plant component content of strawberries may be advantageous for heart health and blood sugar regulation as well as reducing depression [97]. A meta-analysis to evaluate the effects of prebiotics, probiotics, and symbiotics on patients with depression demonstrated the effects of gut microbiota management tools in improving depression [98]. Flaxseed mucilage and gum Arabic could be used to increase the survival of probiotic cultures in kefir without changing its physicochemical properties [99]. Studies show that kefir offers the therapeutic potential of a psych biotic effect. The significant properties of this probiotic beverage (kefir) mainly comprise of antioxidative, immunomodulatory, apoptotic, antitumor, and neuroprotective [100]. Pomegranate juice moderates anxiety and depression [101]. Comprehensive information on the neuroprotective use of ginseng to modulate iron metabolism, reveals its potential to treat Alzheimer's [102]. Brazil nuts are rich on selenium and support the thyroid system.

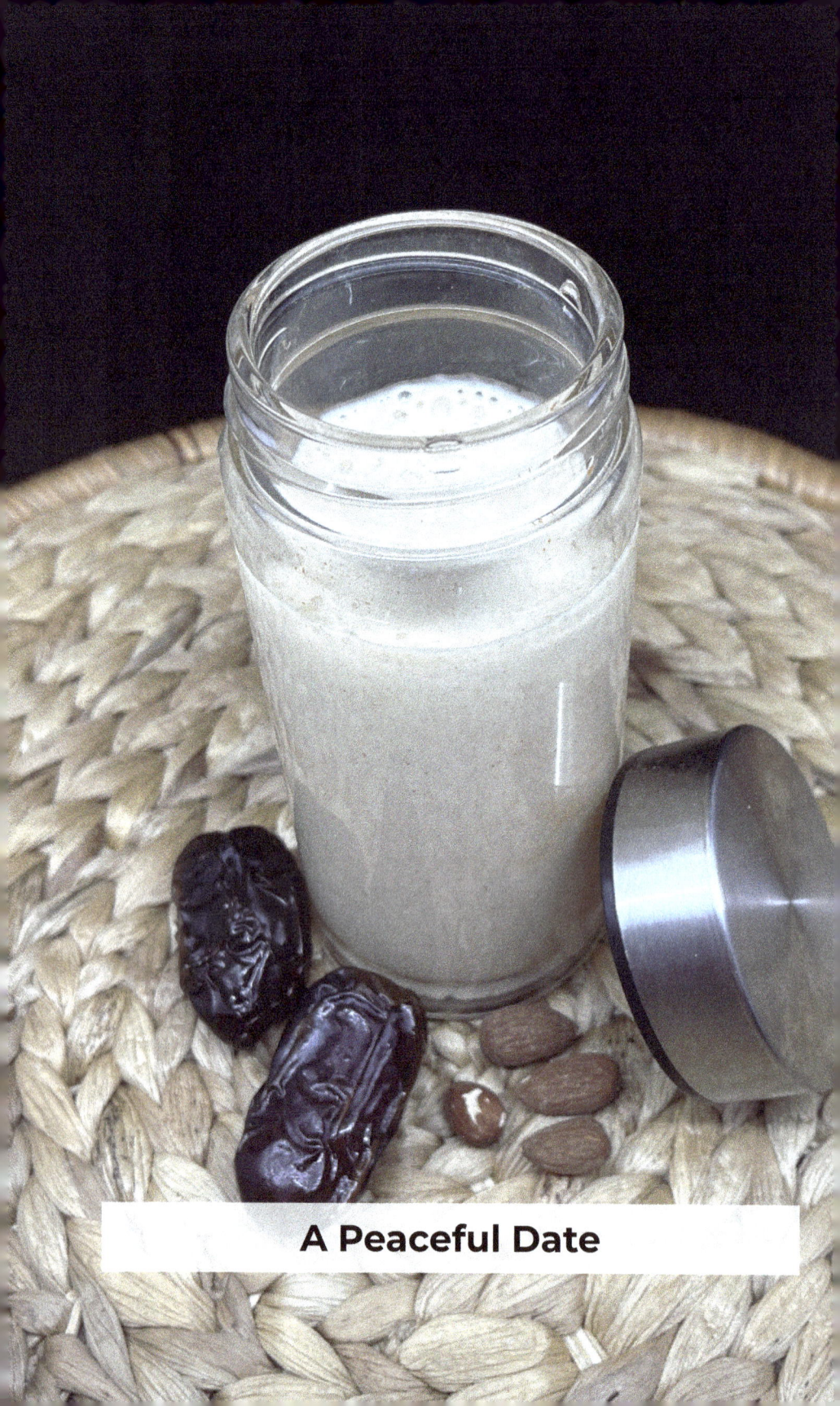
A Peaceful Date

MH2. A Peaceful Date

Embark on a tranquil journey with this blissful smoothie! Almonds and dates support memory while easing anxiety and depression, leaving you feeling suitably serene. The delightful touch of maca and rolled oats add an extra dose of calm to your mind, creating a peaceful oasis you won't ever want to leave. Experience pure serenity in every sip!

INGREDIENTS

🍽 (Serves 1)

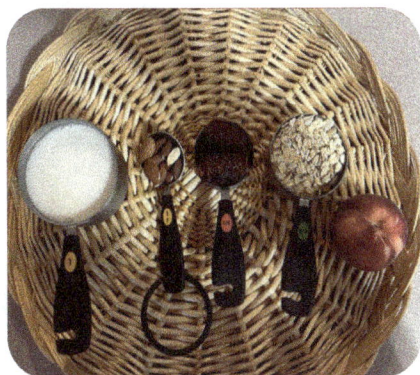

» 12 almonds
» 2 or 3 dates
» 1 ½ cup unsweetened almond milk
» ¼ cup or 2 tablespoons rolled oats
» 1 teaspoon maca
» Half of white peach
» ½ cup of water (if required to thin consistency)

INSTRUCTIONS

1. Remove all seeds from the dates.
2. Soak the dates and almonds in water for 15 minutes.
3. Peel off the almonds. Then, place all dates, almond milk, peach, almonds, and spoons of rolled oats in a blender.
4. Blend until smooth.
5. BON APPETITE!

A Peaceful Date's Ingredients

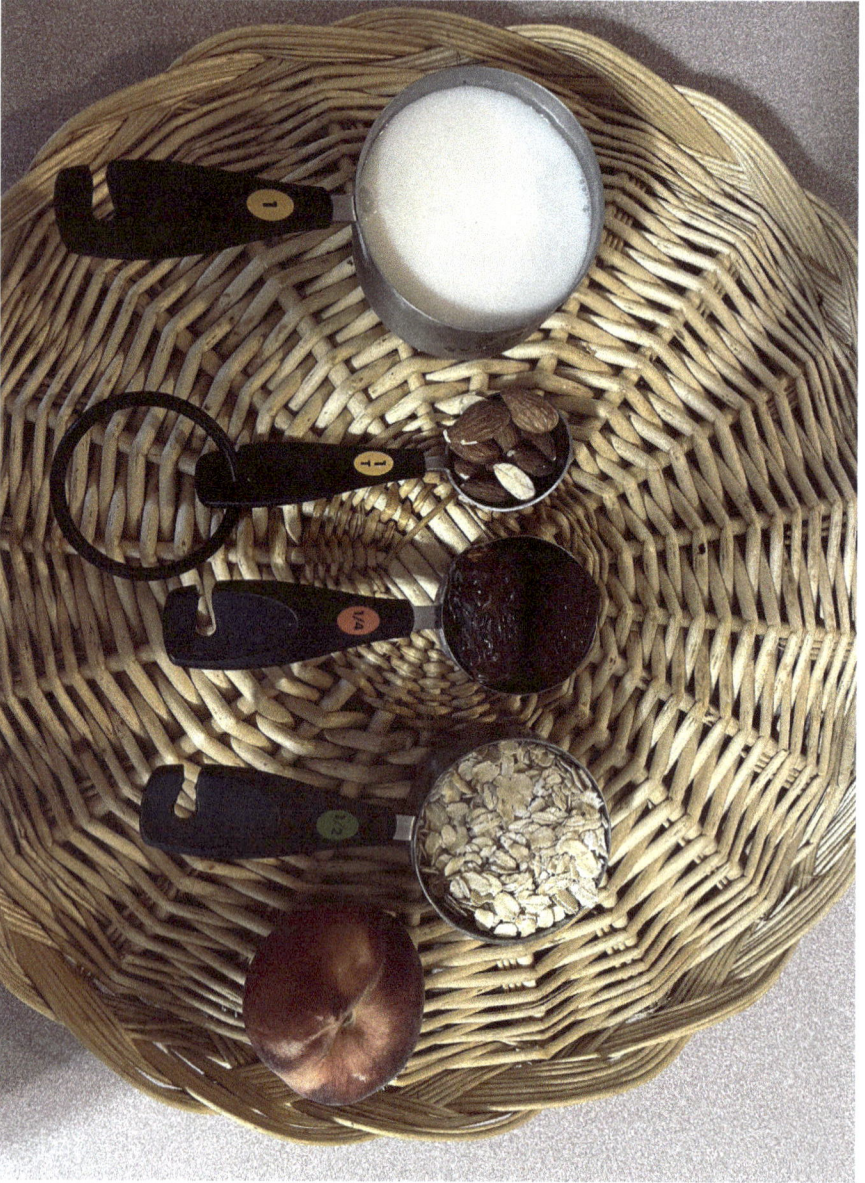

A Peaceful Date nutrition facts and benefits

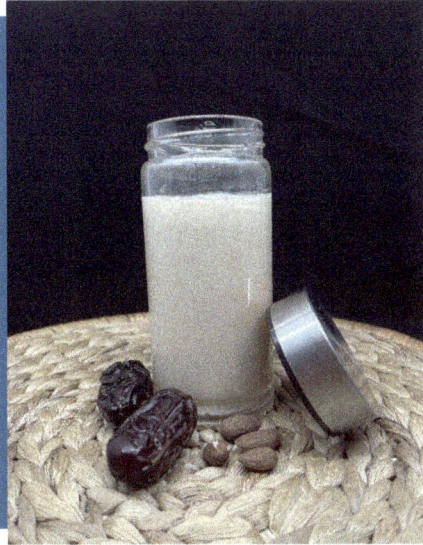

NUTRITION FACTS
(1 serving)

Calories: 231kcals
Carbohydrates: 26.4g
Protein: 6.2g
Fat: 12.4g
Saturated Fat: 0.3g
Cholesterol: 0mg
Sodium: 7.5mg
Potassium: 462mg
Fiber: 4g

HEALTH BENEFITS: The physic-chemical properties of oats, the impact of oats on an array of non-communicable diseases and human microbiome [103]. A diet consisting of 1 serving of almonds per day can help in the reduction of depression and anxiety especially with diabetic patients [104]. Numerous studies have connected higher vitamin E (almonds have vitamin E) intake with reduced risk of cancer, Alzheimer's disease, and heart disease [105]. Maca polysaccharides could enhance the anti-tumor effect, thus suggesting a novel potential immunomodulator in tumor therapy [106]. Dates showed possible beneficial effects concomitant with oxidative stress reduction and increased antioxidant enzymes in Alzheimer's disease transgenic mice model, in addition traditional medicine claims that various components of the phoenix dactylifera (date plant) can be used to treat memory loss, fever, inflammation, loss of consciousness, and nerve disorders [107, 108]. White peach supports immunity.

Almonds: Peeled or not?

The question of eating almonds with or without the skin sparks much debate in regard to their benefits. While raw or roasted almonds are safe to consume, soaked and peeled almonds offer additional advantages.

Almond skin can be hard to digest and contains tannins, which hinder nutrient absorption. Removing the skin can enhance nutrient absorption and ease digestion. Enjoy the best of almonds with this simple switch!

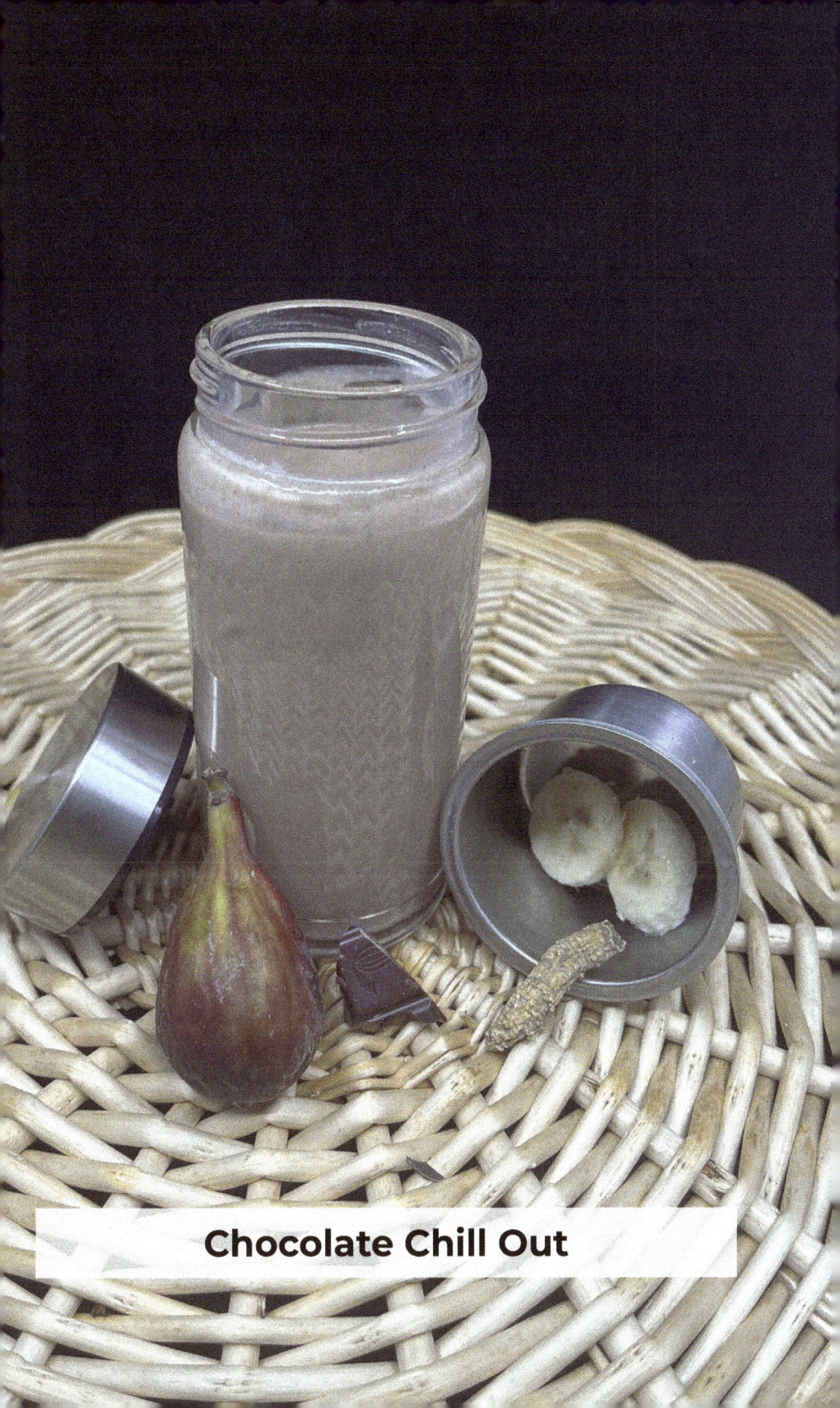

Chocolate Chill Out

MH3. Chocolate Chill Out

Indulge in pure bliss with the Chocolate Chill Out smoothie! Savor the exquisite flavors of figs, banana, and cacao, as your brain enjoys their brain-boosting benefits. And the secret ingredient: maca. With its natural antidepressant effects, maca lifts your spirits, leaving you floating on cloud nine. Treat yourself to this delightful, mood-enhancing blend!

INGREDIENTS

(Serves 1)

» 1 medium size ripe banana
» 3 figs
» 3 squares of dark chocolate (without added sugar)
» 1/4 cup almond yogurt
» 5 walnuts
» 1 tablespoon red Korean ginseng (powder or raw)
» 1 tablespoon maca (optional)
» 1 teaspoon of honey (optional)

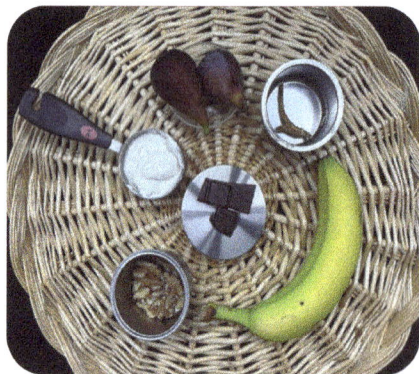

INSTRUCTIONS

1. Add banana chunks, dark chocolate, figs, walnuts, ginseng, and almond yogurt in a high-powered blender.
2. Blend until smooth.
3. Top it with dark chocolate syrup and 1 teaspoon of honey (this step is optional).
4. BON APPETITE!

Chocolate Chill Out's Ingredients

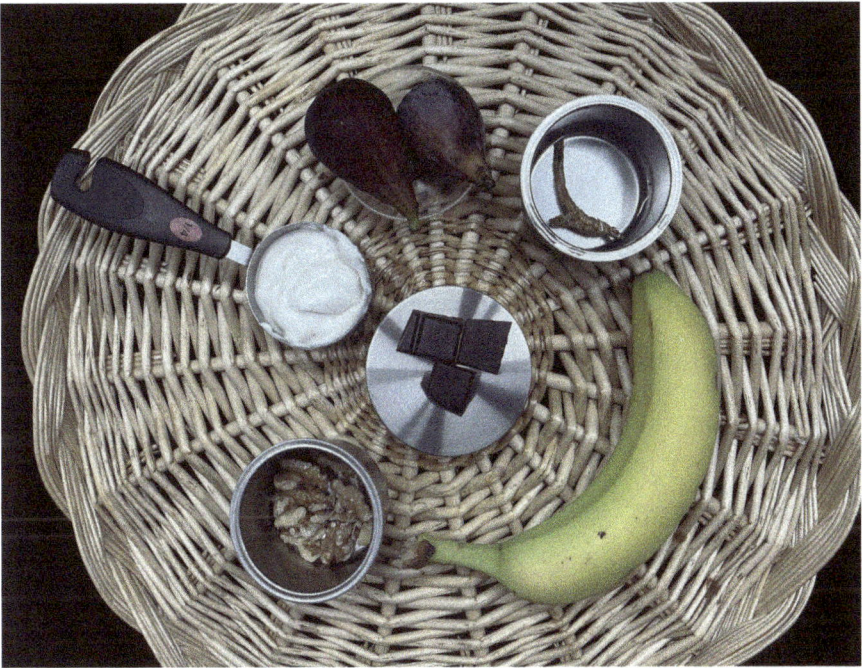

Chocolate Chill Out nutrition facts and benefits

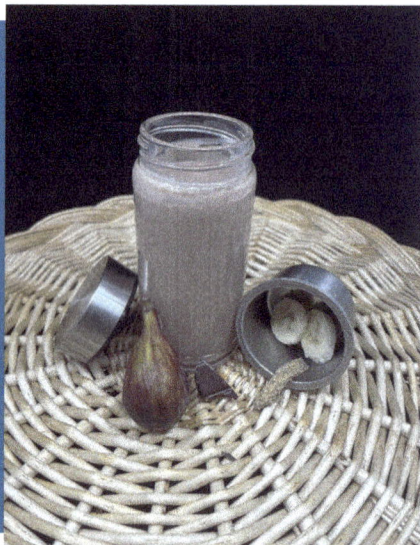

NUTRITION FACTS
(1 serving)

Calories: 267kcals
Carbohydrates: 43.3g
Protein: 3.8g
Fat: 10.9g
Saturated Fat: 3.4 g
Fiber: 4.32g
Cholesterol: 0mg
Sodium: 14.5
Potassium: 636mg

HEALTH BENEFITS: With their rich history dating back 6000 years, figs are one of the oldest known plants to mankind and are a classical fruit in the Mediterranean diet with potential influence on cardiovascular health, diabetes, obesity, and gut/digestive health [109].

Antioxidant flavonoids found in bananas are also far less likely to cause heart disease and brain disorders [52]. Cacao supplementation has been suggested to improve age-related neuronal deficits and the effects of oxidative stress [110]. According to a 2015 study, treatment with 3.3 grammes of maca per day for six weeks improved depressive symptoms compared to a placebo treatment in 29 postmenopausal Chinese women [9]. Korean ginseng boosts liver function and reduces inflammation.

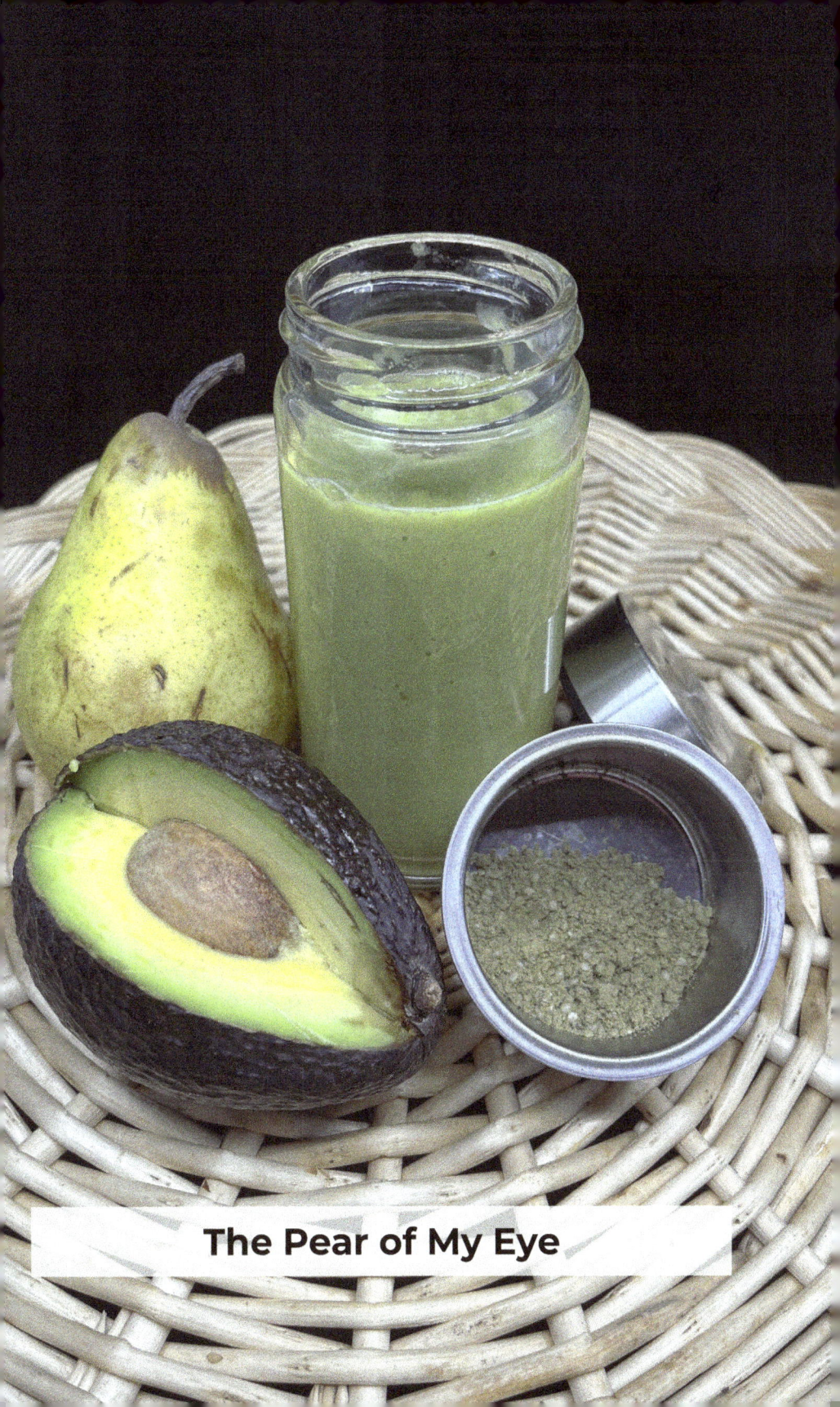

The Pear of My Eye

MH4. The Pear of My Eye

Experience love with The Pear of My Eye smoothie! Dive into a luscious blend of coconut water, pear, mango, matcha, and hemp hearts, whisking you away to a tranquil paradise. This enchanting concoction provides essential nutrients that manage stress and promote a profound sense of calm and well-being, making it your new favorite soul-soother. Embrace the bliss!

INGREDIENTS

🍽 (Serves 2)

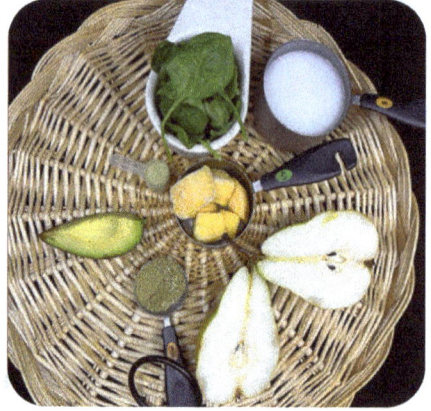

- » 1 ½ cup of spinach
- » 1 cup coconut water
- » 1 pear ripe + cored
- » ½ cup mango frozen
- » ¼ avocado
- » 2 tablespoons hemp hearts
- » 1 scoop of matcha powder (optional)
- » 1 cup of water
- » 1/3 cup of ice cubes or 5 ice cubes

INSTRUCTIONS

1. Blend the spinach and coconut water together until smooth.
2. Add the remaining ingredients and blend again. You can either blend in the hemp hearts or sprinkle them on top.
3. BON APPETITE!

The Pear of My Eye's Ingredients

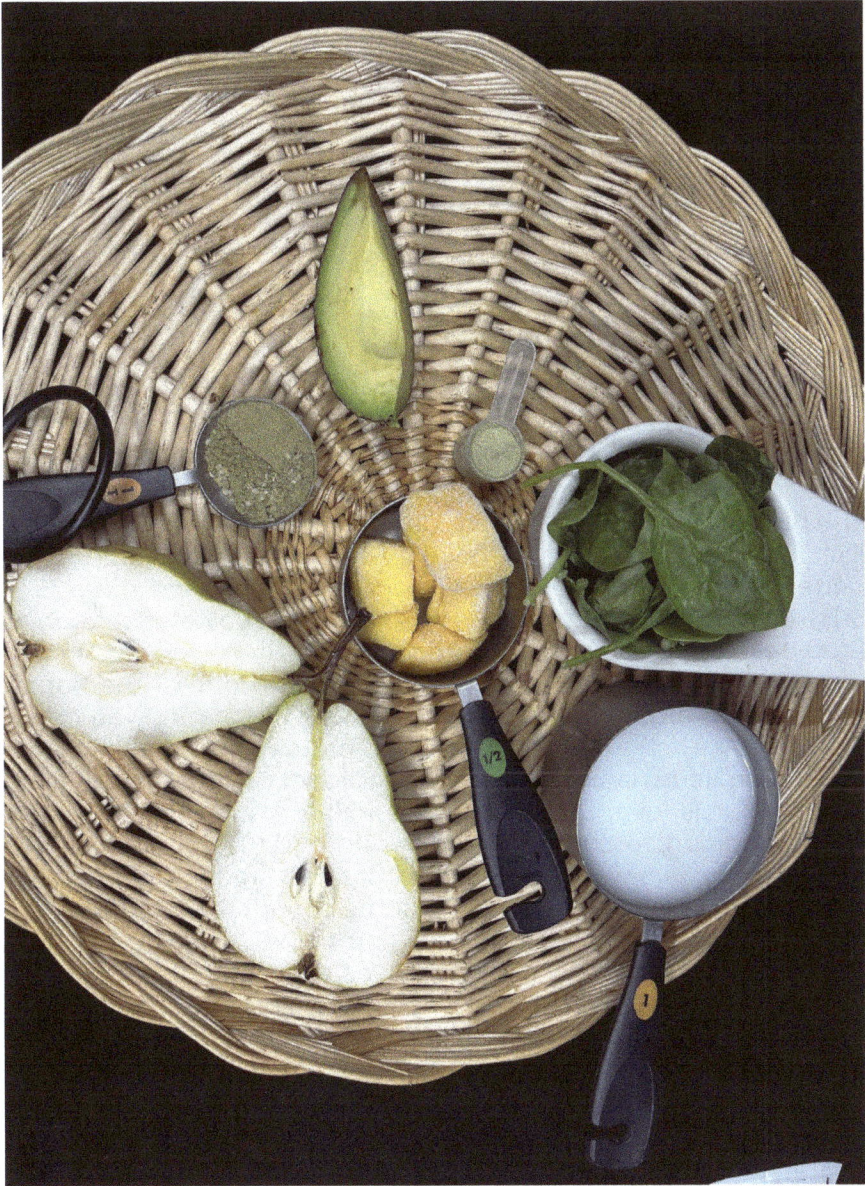

The Pear of My Eye nutrition facts and benefits

NUTRITION FACTS
(1 serving)

Calories: 392kcal
Carbohydrates: 56g
Protein: 12g
Fat: 17g
Saturated Fat: 2g
Cholesterol: 0mg
Sodium: 294mg
Potassium: 1140mg
Fiber: 14g
Sugar: 35g

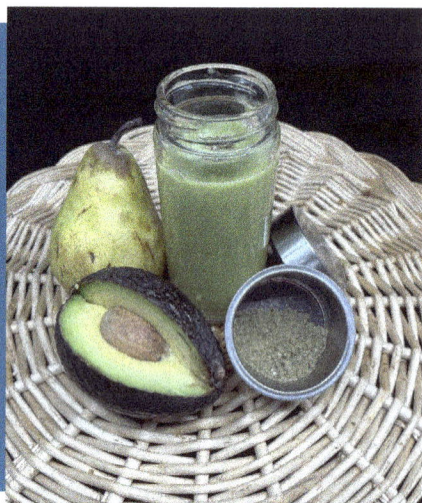

HEALTH BENEFITS: Fruit juice consumption helps with cognitive measures, anxiety, and depression [96]. The greater dietary intake and higher blood levels of antioxidants contained within avocados, like vitamin C and carotenoids, have been associated with better cognitive function, improved heart health, and more [52]. 5-Hydroxyindole acetic acid (5-HIAA) is a metabolite of serotonin. Study results have also shown an increase in 5-HIAA after consuming young coconut water. Serotonin is considered one of the happy hormones. It also helps you manage anger by calming you down [51]. Hemp is a rich source of plant-based protein, and omega-3 and 6 fatty acids. Hemp is also an excellent source of GLA (gamma linoleic acid) and it is ideal to decrease the inflammation of depression [111]. In addition, researchers have shown that the consumption of apples and pears was associated with an 18% reduction in type 2 diabetes [112]. Matcha tea may have some potential effect on weight loss, along with anti-inflammatory properties [113]. In addition, the continued ingestion of matcha was suggested to reduce the anxiety-like behaviors induced by psychological and physiological stresses [114]. Avocado consumption was associated with higher diet quality and intake of plant-based food [115]. The addition of fresh green vegetables such as spinach and kale can enhance the daily supply of micronutrients and significantly increase the bioavailability of bioactive compounds with high antioxidant status [116]. Mango is a nutrient-dense fruit, a study showed that BMI scores, waist circumference, and body weight were significantly lower in male mango consumers when compared with those who did not consume mango [28].

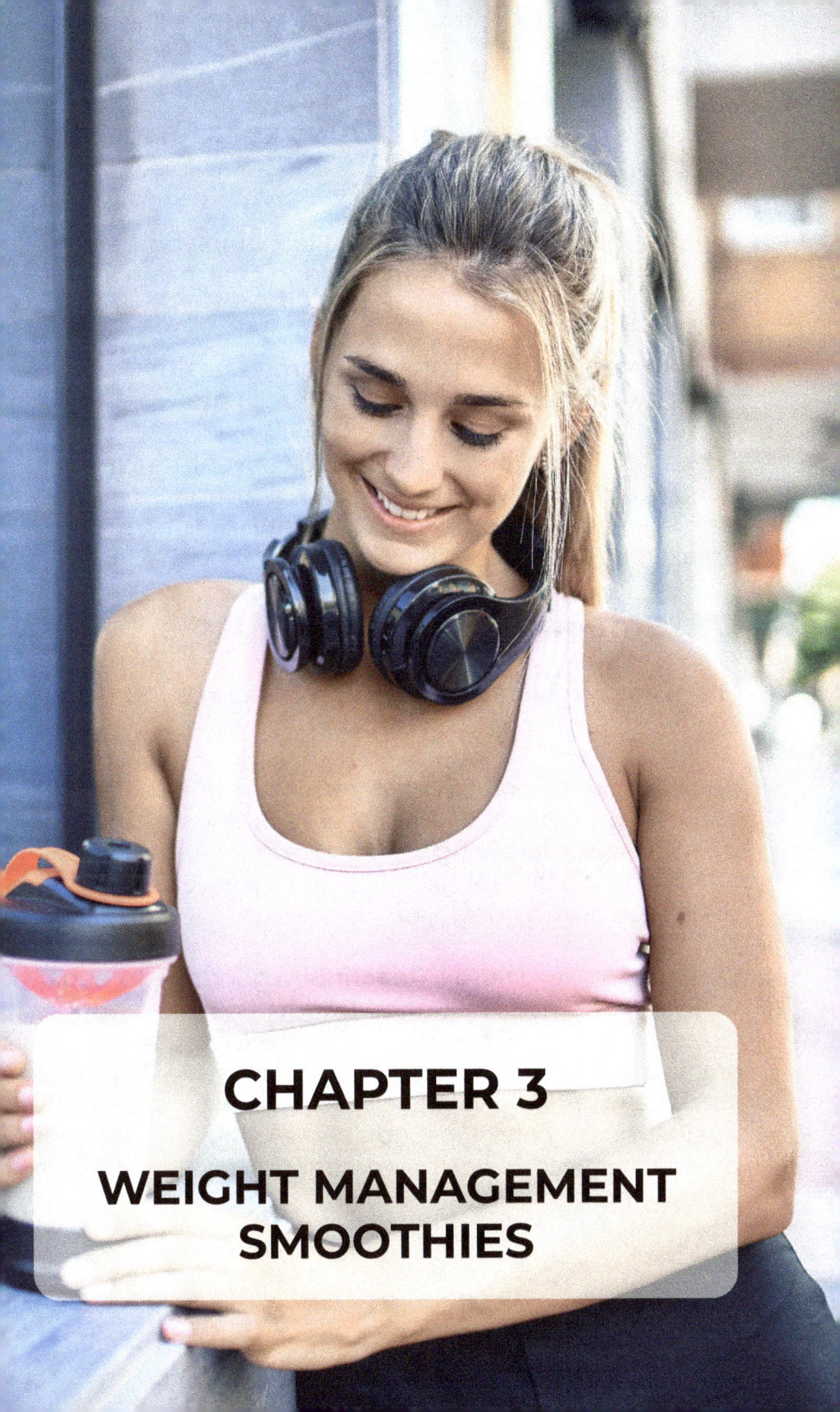

CHAPTER 3

WEIGHT MANAGEMENT SMOOTHIES

Description of smoothies to support weight management.

Weight management is about balancing your weight, eating more healthily, cleansing, and controlling insulin levels for diabetes.

As diabetes and obesity have become a health problem for many, I have divided this into three parts.

Prepare for a thrilling and delicious adventure with my power-packed smoothies designed to fight diabetes, detox your body, and combat obesity! Get ready to be amazed by their incredible benefits:

DB: Smoothies to Fight Diabetes:

DB1. **Dragon Sweet Defense:** Embark on a journey of sweet defense with this extraordinary Dragon Sweet Defense smoothie! Indulge in the magic of dragon fruit and red sweet potato, both renowned for their anti-diabetic properties. The almond milk adds a touch of sweetness while aiding in blood sugar management. This blend is a taste sensation that will leave you feeling energized and in control of your health.

DB2. **No Sugar Daddy Peach:** Say goodbye to sugar worries with my No Sugar Daddy Peach smoothie! Greek yogurt or Greek plant-based yogurt takes the stage, decreasing glucose absorption for a healthier you. The nutritional value of peaches supports the fight against obesity and type 2 diabetes, while the addition of oats helps to lower blood sugar levels. It's a sweet treat without the guilt!

DB3. **Sugar Hangover:** Prepare to beat the sugar hangover with this remarkable smoothie! Cinnamon's magical power helps regulate blood sugar levels, while the berries, spinach, and avocado provide essential fiber and magnesium, thus combating insulin resistance. With the incredible benefits of hemp seeds, you'll be lowering the risk of illnesses, including heart disease and diabetes, in no time!

DX: Detox Smoothies:

DX1. **Bloody Detox:** Revitalize your body with the invigorating Bloody Detox smoothie! Avocado, spinach, green apple, and berries come together to create a powerful detox elixir. Coconut water and pineapple join forces to flush out toxins and support liver health. Beetroot enhances human performance, while ginger aids in gastroenterology health. It's a detoxifying experience like no other!

DX2. **Orange Detox:** Ignite your senses with the zesty Orange Detox smoothie! Oranges, turmeric, and carrots lower blood pressure, reduce inflammation, and protect cells from damage. Ginger adds its spicy twist, while flax seeds provide omega-3 and protein power. Feel the detoxifying effects as you nourish your body and tone your muscles.

DX3. **Parsley Purification:** Experience the purification benefits of the Parsley Purification smoothie! Moringa protects you with its nutritional goodness, while the addition of avocado, pineapple, and collard greens support your healthy diet. The parsley's potent properties are balanced with a delightful mix of flavors that will leave you feeling refreshed and renewed. Meanwhile, matcha provides a rich flavor that regulates the microbiota.

WM: Smoothies to Fight Obesity:

WM1. **Skinny Pineapple:** Discover the secrets of weight management with Skinny Pineapple smoothie! Pineapple, cultured low-fat milk probiotics, nuts, and spinach come together to protect your microbiota and support metabolic health. Sip your way to a slimmer, healthier you!

WM2. **Mango Hunger Tamer:** Quell your hunger pangs with this tantalizing smoothie! Mango and raspberries work their magic, providing nutrient-dense and fiber-rich goodness. Add a scoop of your favorite protein, whether it's whey or collagen, and the calming effects of maca to complete this satisfying blend.

WM3. **Resistant Starch:** Discover the power of resistant starch with Resistant Starch smoothie! Cucumbers, spinach, and fruits like pineapple, unripe banana, kiwi, and avocado provide fiber and essential nutrients that support weight loss. Spirulina's protein brings a nutrient-dense boost, supplying your body with essential amino acids. Prepare to conquer your appetite and achieve your weight loss goals!

With these thrilling smoothies by your side, you'll be ready to take on the world and achieve your healthiest, happiest self! Cheers to a life of vitality and wellness!

SHOPPING LIST FOR WEIGHT MANAGEMENT

Berries: Blueberries, strawberries, raspberries

Fruits: Banana, pineapple, mango, kiwi, green apple, avocado, dragon fruit, white peach, orange

Greens: Spinach, collard greens, mint, parsley

Vegetables: Sweet potato, purple sweet potato, red beet, carrot

Roots: Ginger, turmeric

Additives: Flax seeds grounded, chia seeds, hemp seeds, cinnamon powder, black pepper, cayenne pepper, matcha powder, vanilla, spirulina powder, maca powder, moringa powder.

Liquid: Unsweetened almond milk, coconut water, sugar free Greek or Greek plant based yogurt, lemon juice, kefir or probiotic

Nuts: Almonds, pecans, walnuts

Others: Collagen powder, whey powder (if you are not allergic to milk), rolled oats

SMOOTHIES TO FIGHT DIABETES

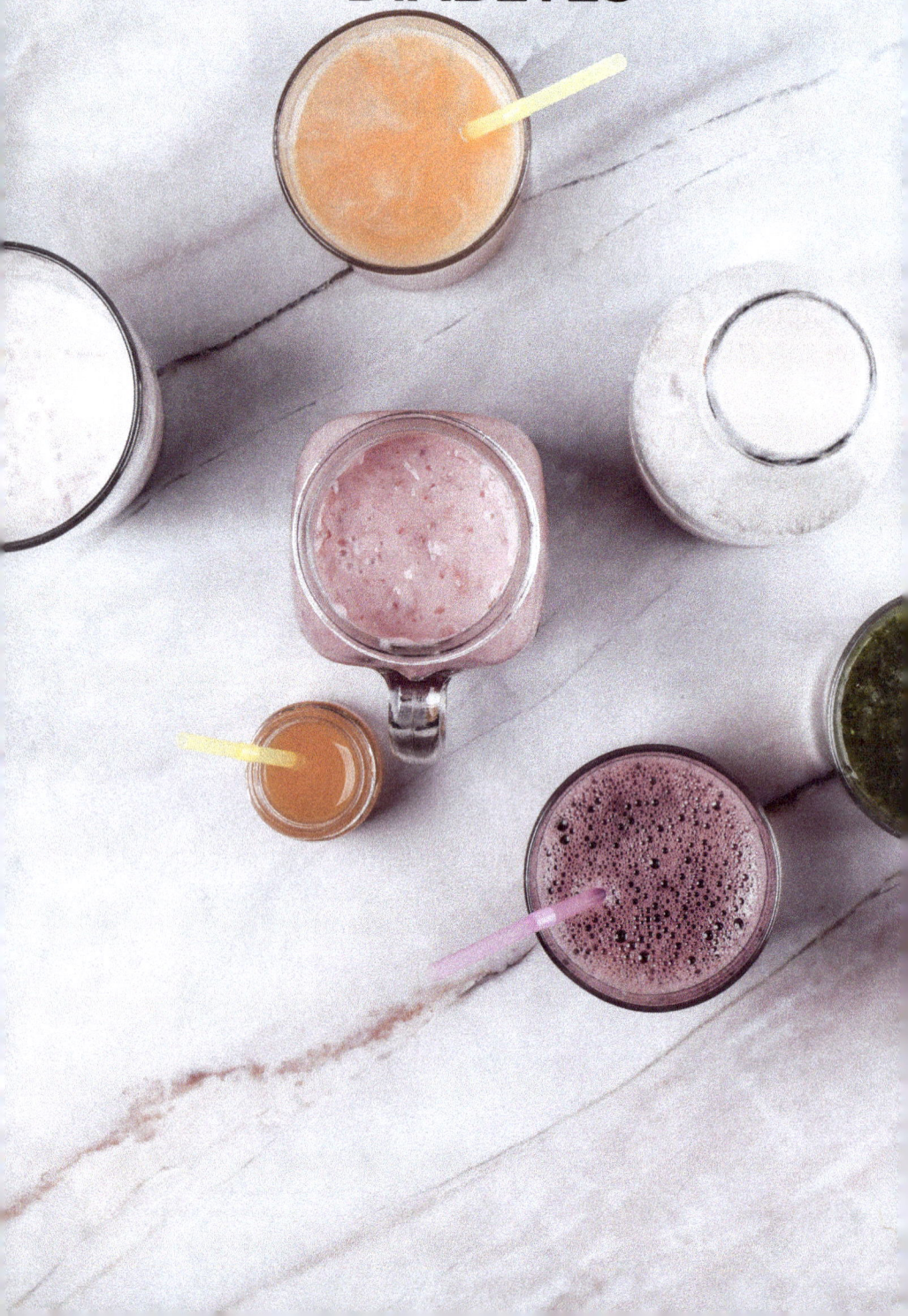

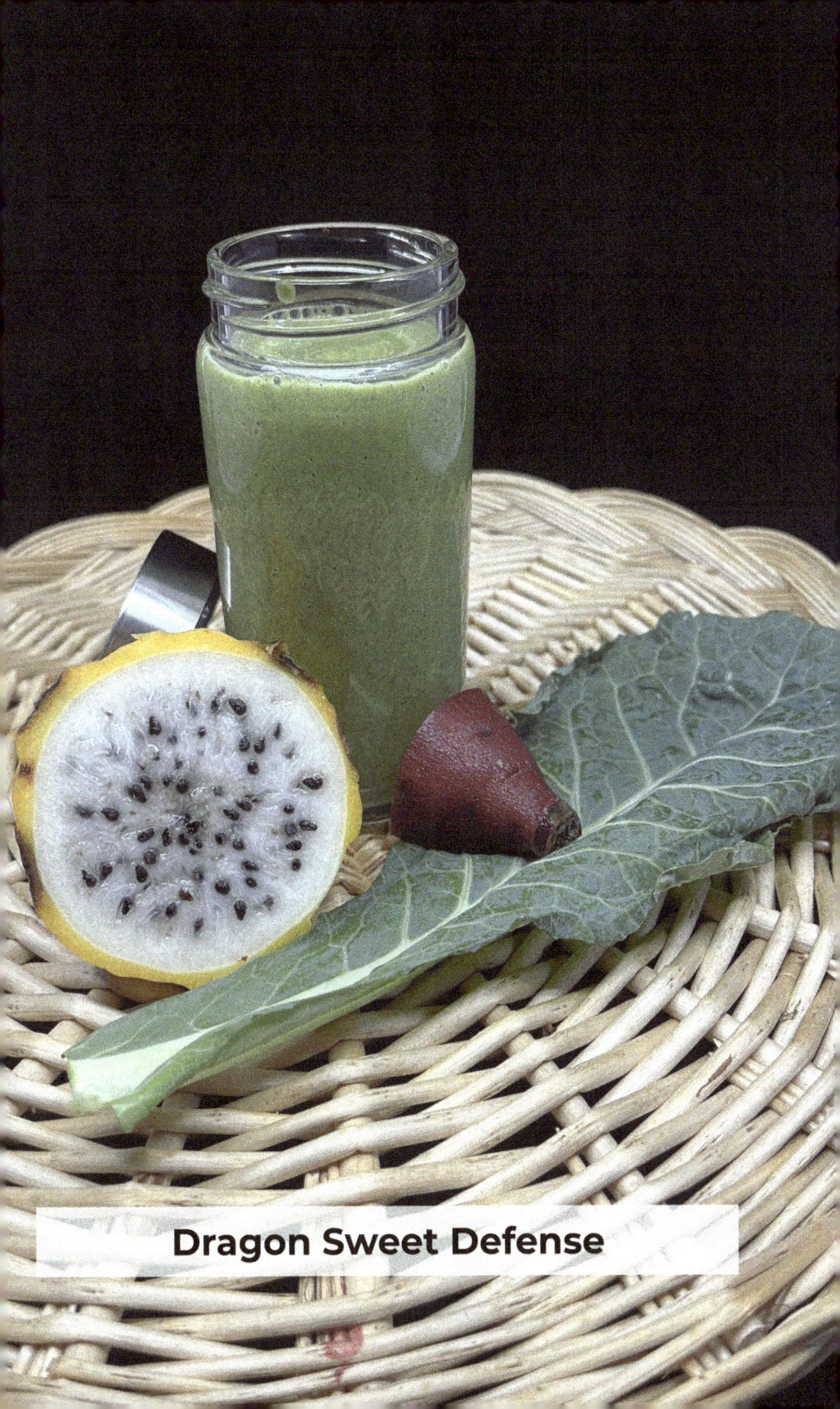
Dragon Sweet Defense

DB1. Dragon Sweet Defense

Embark on a sweet defense journey with the extraordinary Dragon Sweet Defense smoothie! Discover the magic of dragon fruit and red sweet potato, known for their anti-diabetic properties. Almond milk adds a touch of sweetness and aids in blood sugar management. This taste sensation will leave you energized and in control of your health.

INGREDIENTS

🛎 (Serves 2)

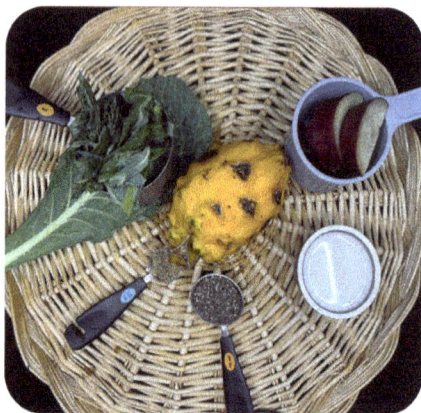

- » 1 cup unsweetened almond milk
- » 1 dragon fruit peeled or 1 cup of frozen dragon fruit
- » 1 cup collard greens
- » 1 cup raw sweet potato with peel. This is equivalent to 1/2 medium sweet potato (you may boil for 5 minutes to soften it)
- » 1 tablespoon chia seeds
- » ½ tablespoon flaxseeds (or flaxseeds in powder)
- » 1/2 cup of water
- » 5 ice cubes

INSTRUCTIONS

1. How to peel a dragon fruit? Well, you don't peel it! You cut it in half, and with a spoon take the meat out and then put the meat into the blender.
2. Blend all of the ingredients together. BON APPETITE!

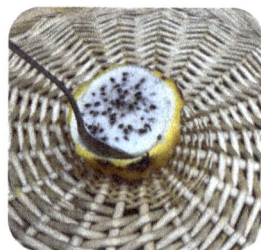

Take the meat with a spoon!

Dragon Sweet Defense's Ingredients

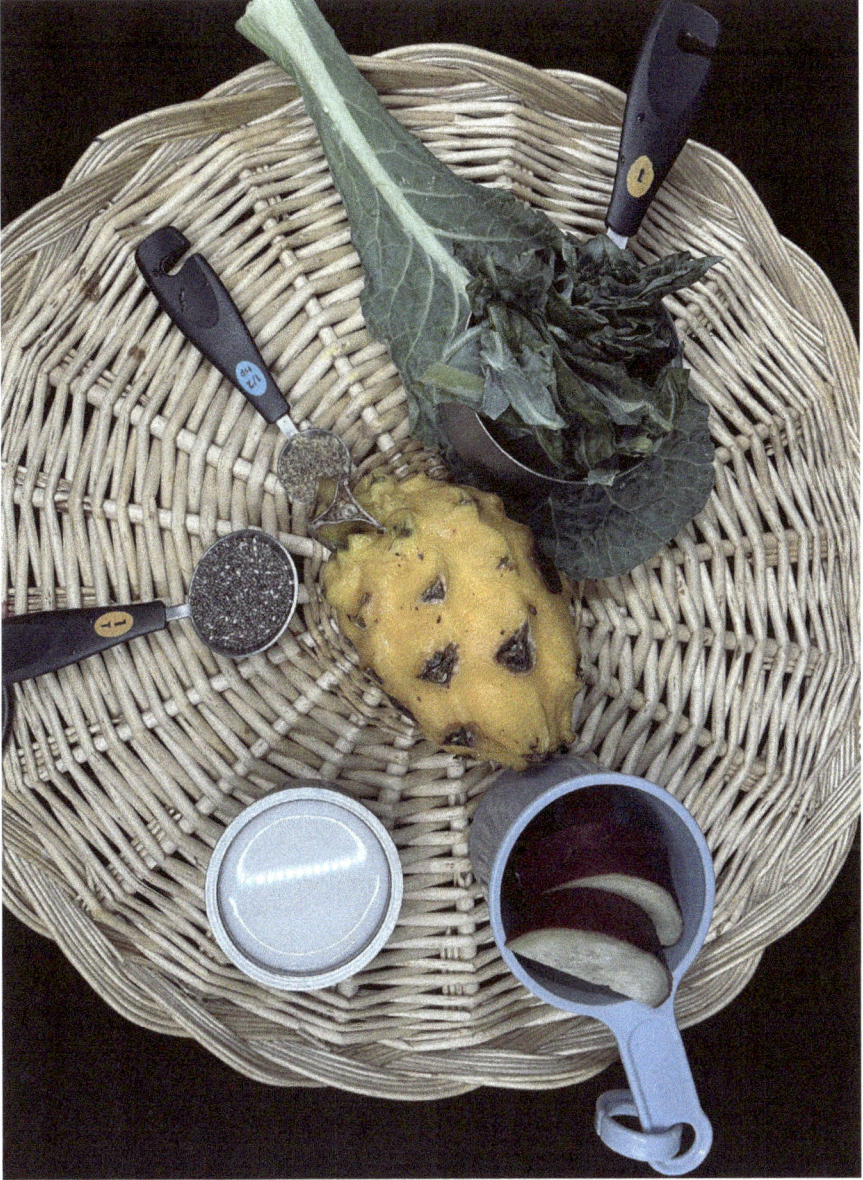

Dragon Sweet Defense nutrition facts and benefits

NUTRITION FACTS (1 serving)

Calories: 404kcal
Carbohydrates: 38g
Protein: 12g
Fat: 26g
Saturated Fat: 1g
Cholesterol: 0mg
Sodium: 257mg
Potassium: 329mg
Fiber: 16g
Sugar: 16g

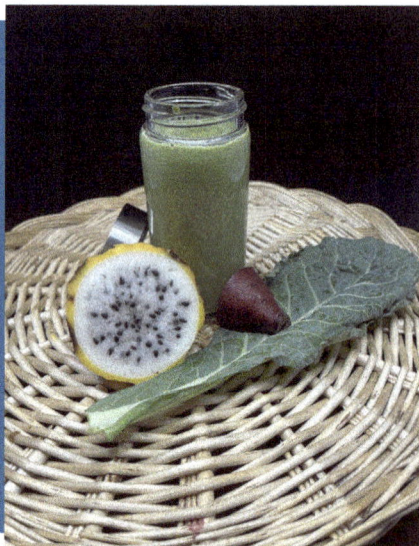

HEALTH BENEFITS: Several studies show that almond consumption results in improved blood sugar management in persons with type 2 diabetes, which has been linked by a reputable source [117]. Animal studies suggest that chia seeds may enhance insulin sensitivity, which is very encouraging. After eating, this may aid in stabilizing blood sugar levels [118]. Red dragon fruit (Hylocereus polyrhizus, F.A.C. Weber Britton and Rose) has been reported to have various biological activities such as antimicrobial, anti-hypercholesterolemia, anti-diabetes mellitus, cardiovascular risk reduction, health supplement, and melanoma cell inhibitory [119]. Sweet potato has been found to control hyperglycemia. Hyperglycemia is a condition with high glucose levels that may result in dyslipidemia. In severe cases, this alteration may lead to diabetic retinopathy [120].

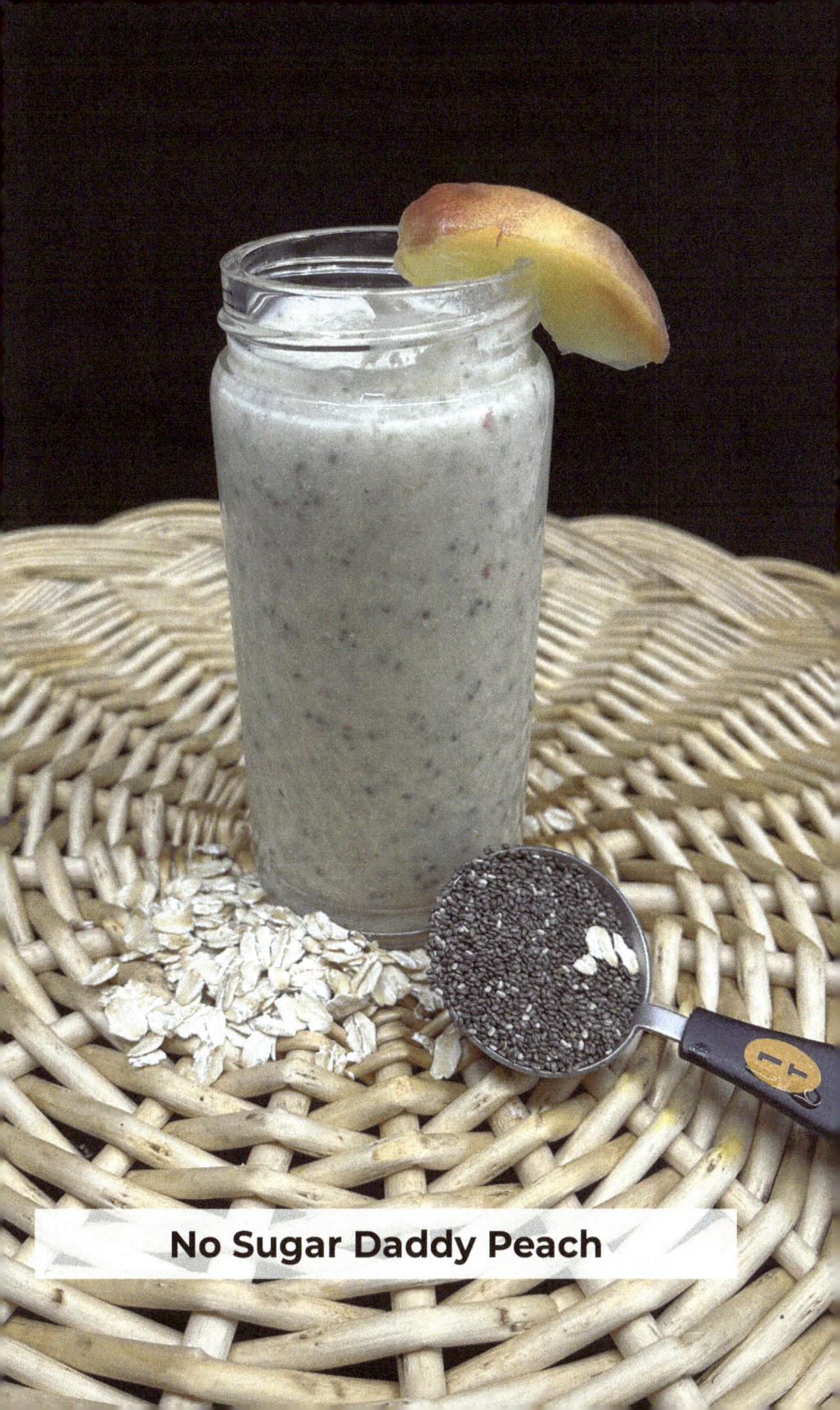

No Sugar Daddy Peach

DB2. No Sugar Daddy Peach

Bid farewell to sugar worries with the No Sugar Daddy Peach smoothie! Greek yogurt or Greek plant-based yogurt takes the stage, reducing glucose absorption for a healthier you. The nutritional value of peaches support the fight against obesity and type 2 diabetes, while oats aid in lowering blood sugar levels. Enjoy a guilt-free sweet treat!

INGREDIENTS

(Serves 1)

» 1/4 cup old fashioned oats or rolled oats
» 1 tablespoon sunflower butter or creamy peanut butter
» ½ banana
» 1 white peach
» ½ cup unsweetened plain Greek yogurt or vanilla unsweetened Greek plant-based yogurt
» 1 teaspoon chia seeds (optional)
» ½ cup water + 5 ice cubes

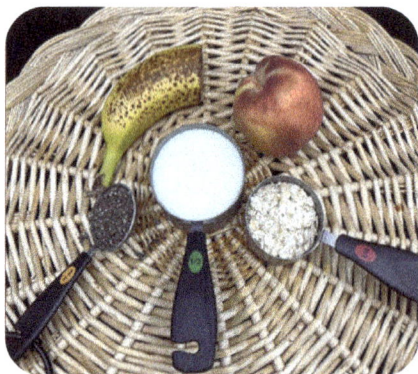

INSTRUCTIONS

1. Add all of the ingredients to a blender.
2. Blend for 30 seconds or until the smoothie is creamy and lump free.
3. Pour into a glass and garnish with banana slices and oats if desired. Serve immediately or place in the refrigerator until you're ready to consume.

No Sugar Daddy Peach's Ingredients

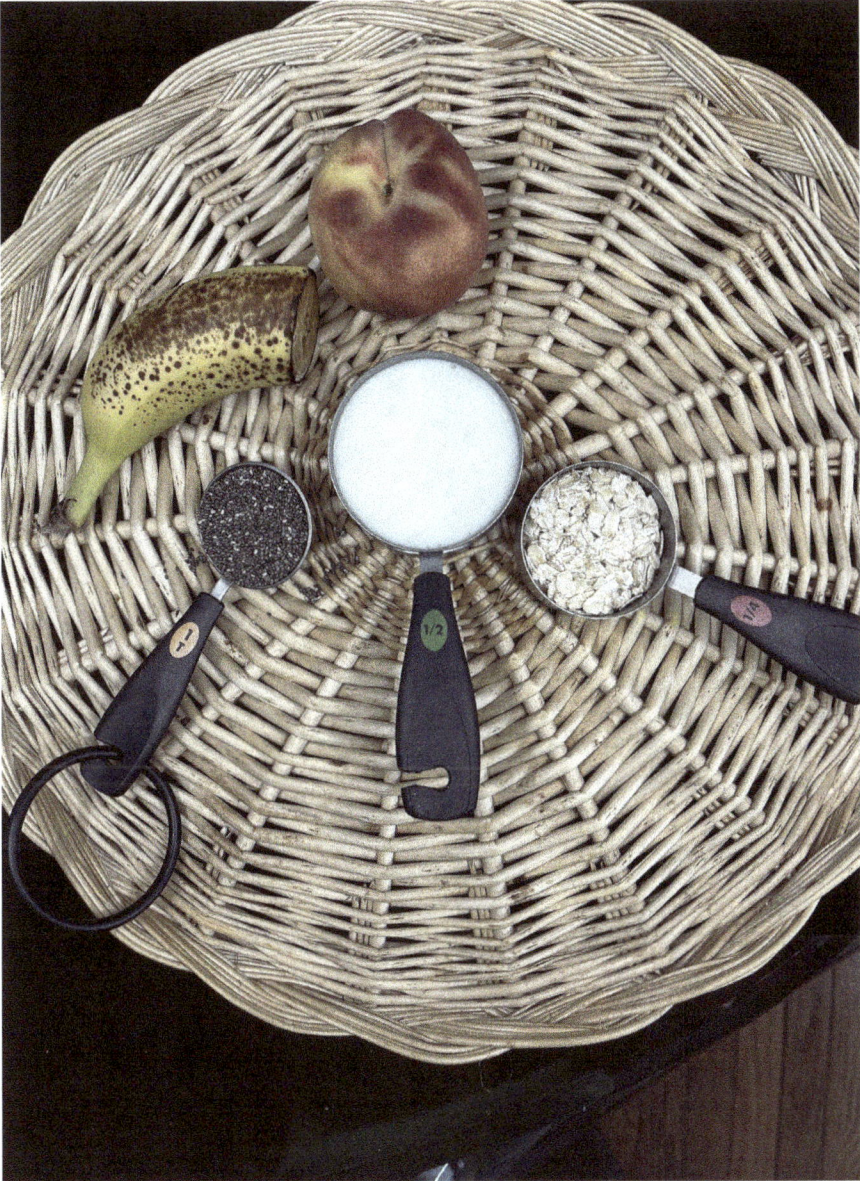

No Sugar Daddy Peach nutrition facts and benefits

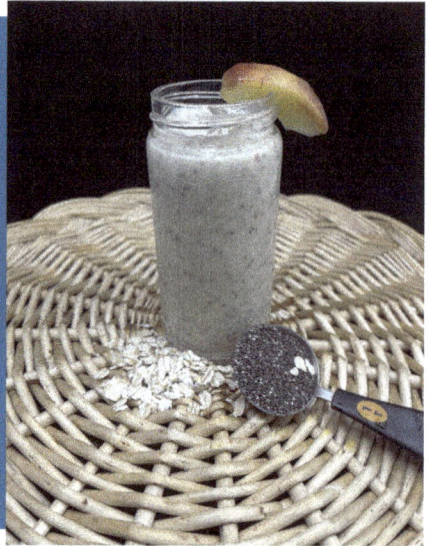

NUTRITION FACTS
(1 serving)

Calories: 423kcal
Carbohydrates: 50g
Protein: 16g
Fat: 20g
Saturated Fat: 4g
Cholesterol: 0mg
Sodium: 208mg
Potassium: 869mg
Fiber: 8g
Sugar: 20g

HEALTH BENEFITS: Oats may help to lower blood sugar levels, especially in people who are overweight or have type 2 diabetes. The beta-glucan in both oats and barley may also improve insulin sensitivity [121]. Animal studies suggest that chia seeds may enhance insulin sensitivity, which is encouraging. After eating, this may aid in stabilizing blood sugar levels [118]. Greek-style yogurt with the encapsulated hydrolysates has shown the ability to inhibit enzymes related to carbohydrate metabolism that could help decrease glucose absorption for type 2 diabetes patients [122]. Peaches have a varied chemical composition and nutritional value, especially with high inhibitory potential against digestive enzymes linked to obesity and type 2 diabetes, strongly determined by the cultivar [123].

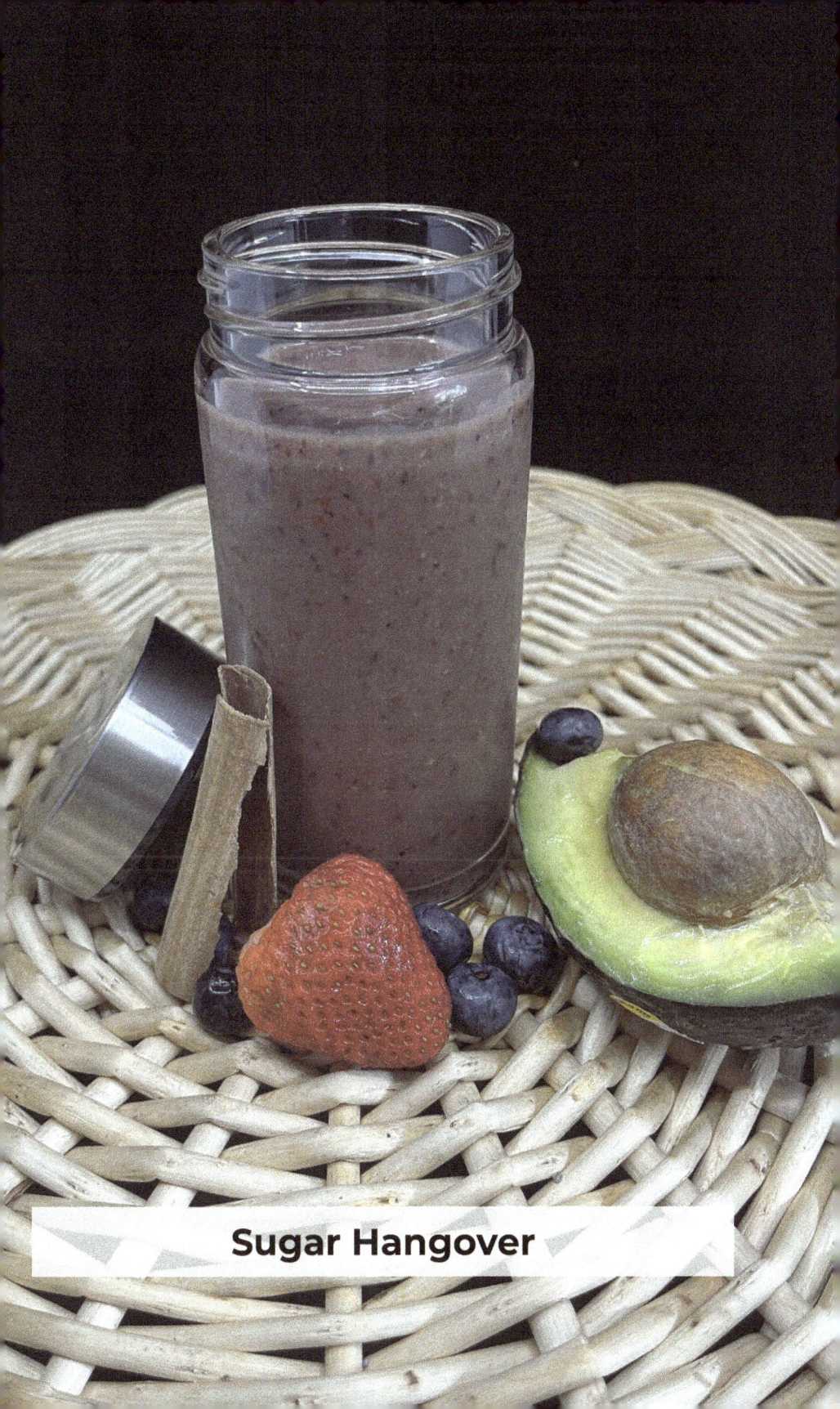

Sugar Hangover

DB3. Sugar Hangover

Get ready to conquer the sugar hangover with this remarkable smoothie! Cinnamon regulates blood sugar levels, while the blend of berries, spinach, and avocado supply essential fiber and magnesium, thus combating insulin resistance. Enjoy the incredible benefits of hemp seeds, lowering the risk of illnesses like heart disease and diabetes. Embrace a healthier you in no time!

INGREDIENTS

(Serves 1)

» ½ cup almond milk unsweetened
» ⅛ cup of lemon juice (equivalent to the juice of half a lemon)
» ½ cup fresh baby spinach
» ¼ medium avocado sliced
» ½ cup frozen (or not) blueberries
» ¼ cup frozen (or raw) strawberries
» ½ teaspoon hemp seeds
» ¼ teaspoon cinnamon powder
» ½ cup water

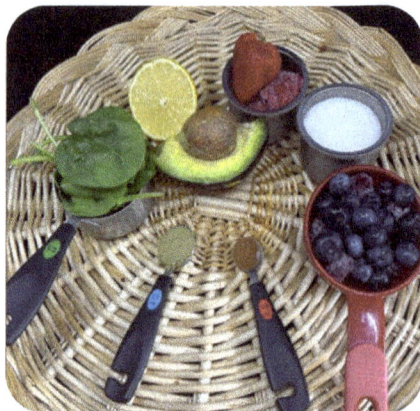

INSTRUCTIONS

1. Gather all the smoothie ingredients and get your blender ready. Place all the ingredients into the blender in the following order - so that you don't have to stop and stir all the time or end up with a chunky smoothie, which is not fun!
2. Put in the almond milk, lemon juice (this is a berry smoothie game changer – don't' skip out on this one) and baby spinach. After that, add the avocado, frozen berries, hemp seeds (let's take a break from the usual chia seeds and amp up the protein) and cinnamon powder.

3. Blend the ingredients on a high speed until smooth and creamy. This will take about 50-60 seconds. Taste and adjust the consistency or flavoring if needed. Pour the smoothie into the glasses. Serve and enjoy immediately!
4. BON APPETITE!

Sugar Hangover nutrition facts and benefits

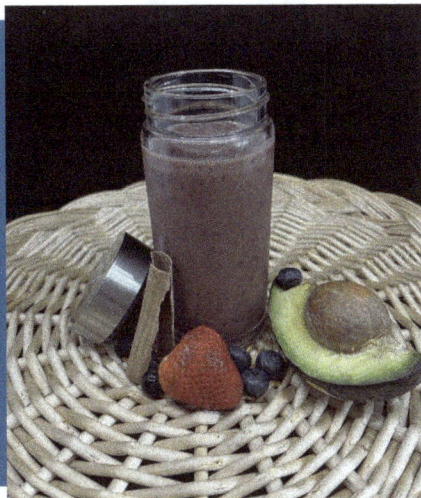

NUTRITION FACTS (1 serving)

Calories: 120kcal
Carbohydrates: 15g
Protein: 5g
Fat: 5g
Saturated Fat: 1g
Cholesterol: 0mg
Sodium: 176mg
Potassium: 201mg
Fiber: 4g
Sugar: 9g

HEALTH BENEFITS: Almond consumption and improved blood sugar management in persons with type 2 diabetes are linked by a reputable source [117]. They discovered that avocados do not significantly impact blood sugar levels. Part of what makes avocados a good choice for people with diabetes is that, although they are low in carbs, they are high in fiber. Furthermore, strawberries are a good source of fiber. Fresh, whole strawberries have about 3 grams (g) of fiber per cup, or about 13% of the daily required amount. Magnesium and vitamin C are two more crucial elements and vitamins that can be found in strawberries. According to a study, magnesium may help with insulin resistance, lowering the risk of type 2 diabetes and enhancing diabetic management [124]. Also associated with reduced inflammation is the gamma-linolenic acid found in hemp seeds, which may lower the risk of illnesses including heart disease, and diabetes [125]. Clinical studies revealed that cinnamon has an anti-inflammatory impact as well, which may be helpful for those with diabetes. Based on in vitro and in vivo investigations, cinnamon appears to cause an insulin-mimicking impact and an increase in enzyme activity that regulate glucose metabolism in tissues [126].

Sugar Hangover's Ingredients

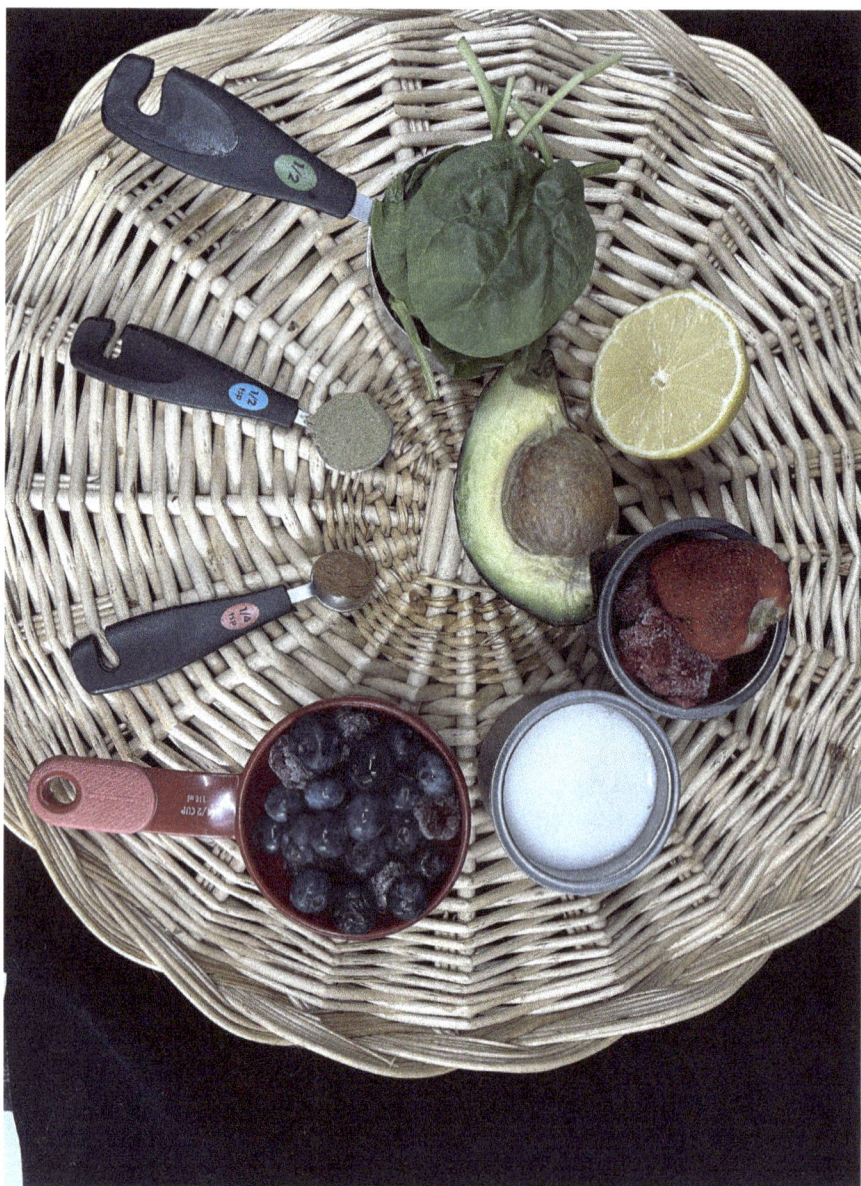

DETOX SMOOTHIES

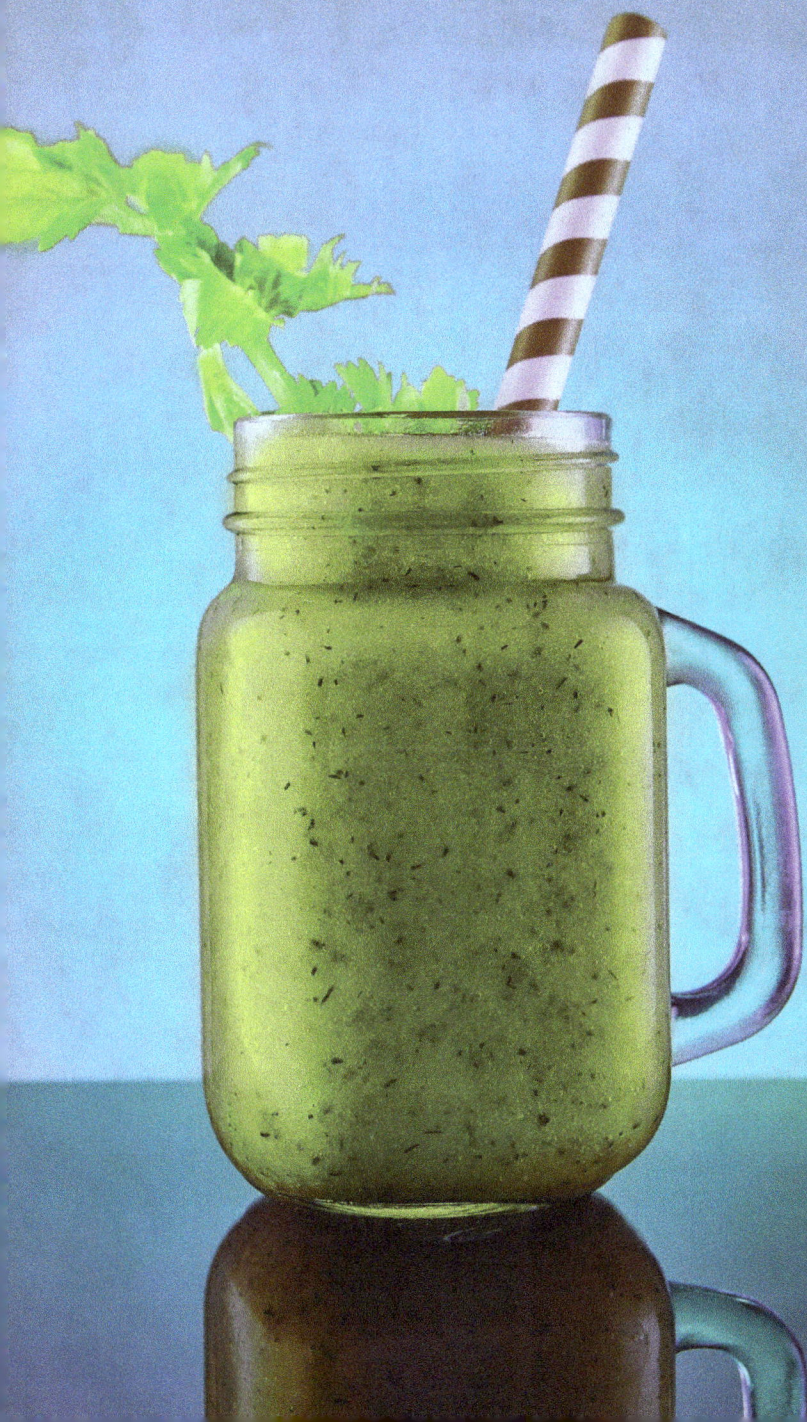

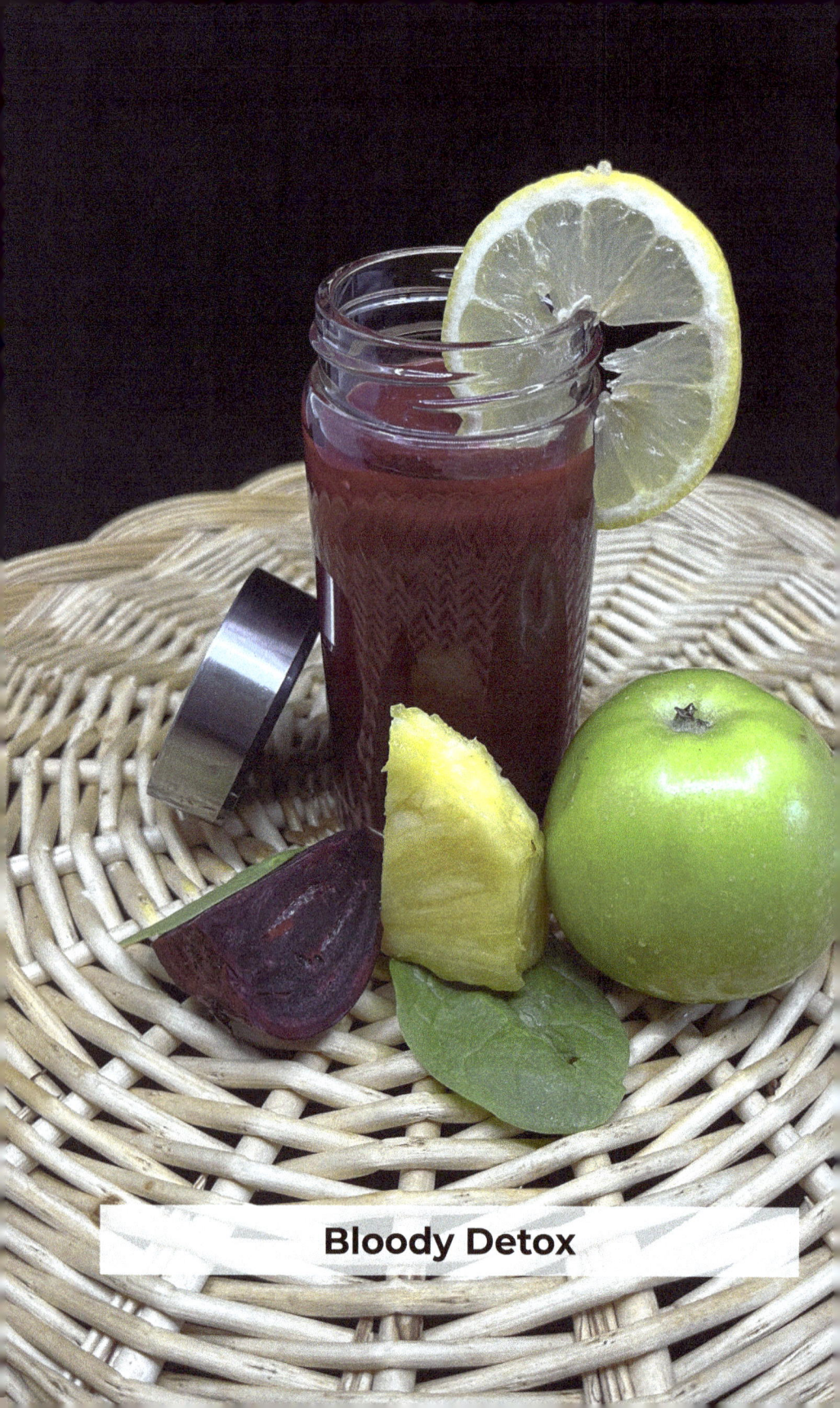

Bloody Detox

DX1. Bloody Detox

Revitalize with my invigorating Bloody Detox smoothie! Avocado, spinach, green apple, and berries form a potent detox elixir. Coconut water and pineapple work to flush out toxins in support of liver health. Beetroot enhances performance, while ginger aids gastroenterology health. An unparalleled detoxifying experience awaits!

INGREDIENTS

🍽 (Serves 2)

» 1 cup raw coconut water or filtered water, add more as needed
» 1 medium green apple, skin on, cored and diced
» 1 small raw red beet, peeled and diced (grated for conventional blenders)
» 1 cup frozen strawberries
» 1 cup frozen pineapple
» ¼ small avocado pitted and peeled
» 1 cup baby spinach
» 1 tablespoon fresh lemon juice
» 1 teaspoon of ginger
» ½ cup of water + 5 ice cubes
» A pinch of cayenne pepper (optional)

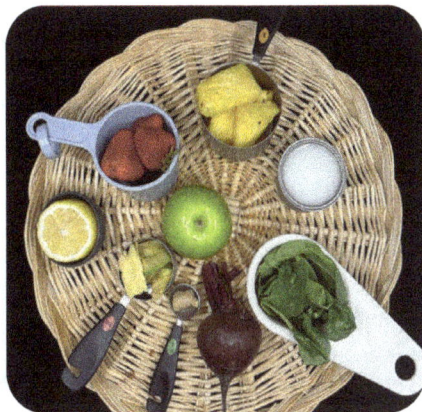

INSTRUCTIONS

1. Throw all the ingredients into your blender, and blast on high for 30 to 60 seconds until smooth and creamy.
2. Pour into glasses and serve immediately.
3. BON APPETITE!

Bloody Detox's Ingredients

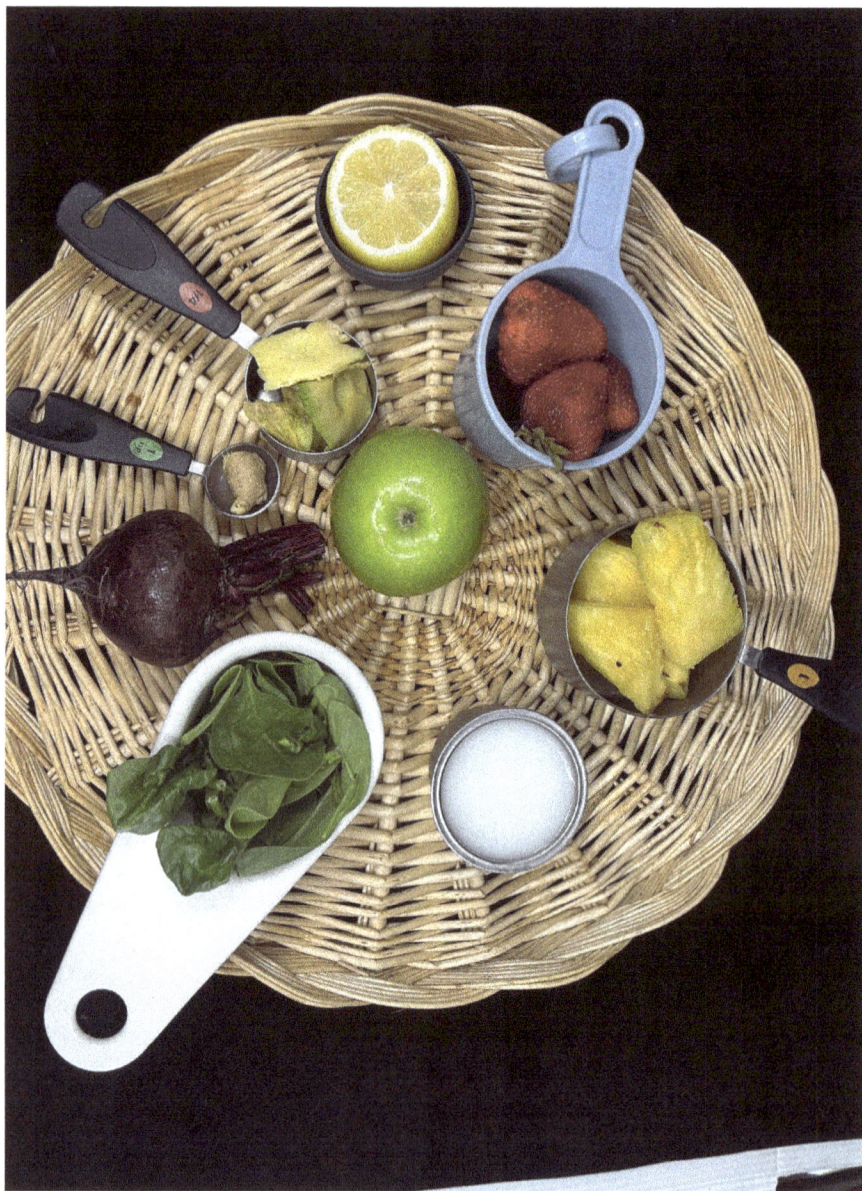

Bloody Detox nutrition facts and benefits

**NUTRITION FACTS
(1 serving)**

Calories: 210kcal
Carbohydrates: 36g
Protein: 4g
Fat: 8g
Saturated Fat: 1g
Cholesterol: 0mg
Sodium: 183mg
Potassium: 1022mg
Fiber: 10g
Sugar: 21g

HEALTH BENEFITS: Pineapples contain other micronutrients, such as copper, thiamine, and vitamin B6, which are essential for healthy metabolism [10]. If your liver gets overloaded as a result of the following conditions, you may develop a condition known as nonalcoholic fatty liver disease: a bad diet, exposure to hazardous chemicals, excessive alcohol consumption and sedentary kind of life. Betaine, an antioxidant, may help prevent or lessen fatty liver deposits. Betaine might also shield poisons from your liver. Another 2014 study discovered that coconut water treatment significantly reduced oxidative stress in damaged rat livers when compared to livers that did not get treatment [127]. Cayenne pepper includes other healthy substances, such as carotenoids and flavonoids, which have anti-inflammatory and antioxidant qualities, in addition to capsaicin [128]. Beetroot juice is a food high in nitrate and is associated with cardiometabolic health benefits. Recent clinical trials have shown that beetroot supplementation improves human performance [129, 130]. Ginger root extract improved glucose homeostasis by improving intestinal integrity and mitochondrial dysfunction of gastroenterology health [131].

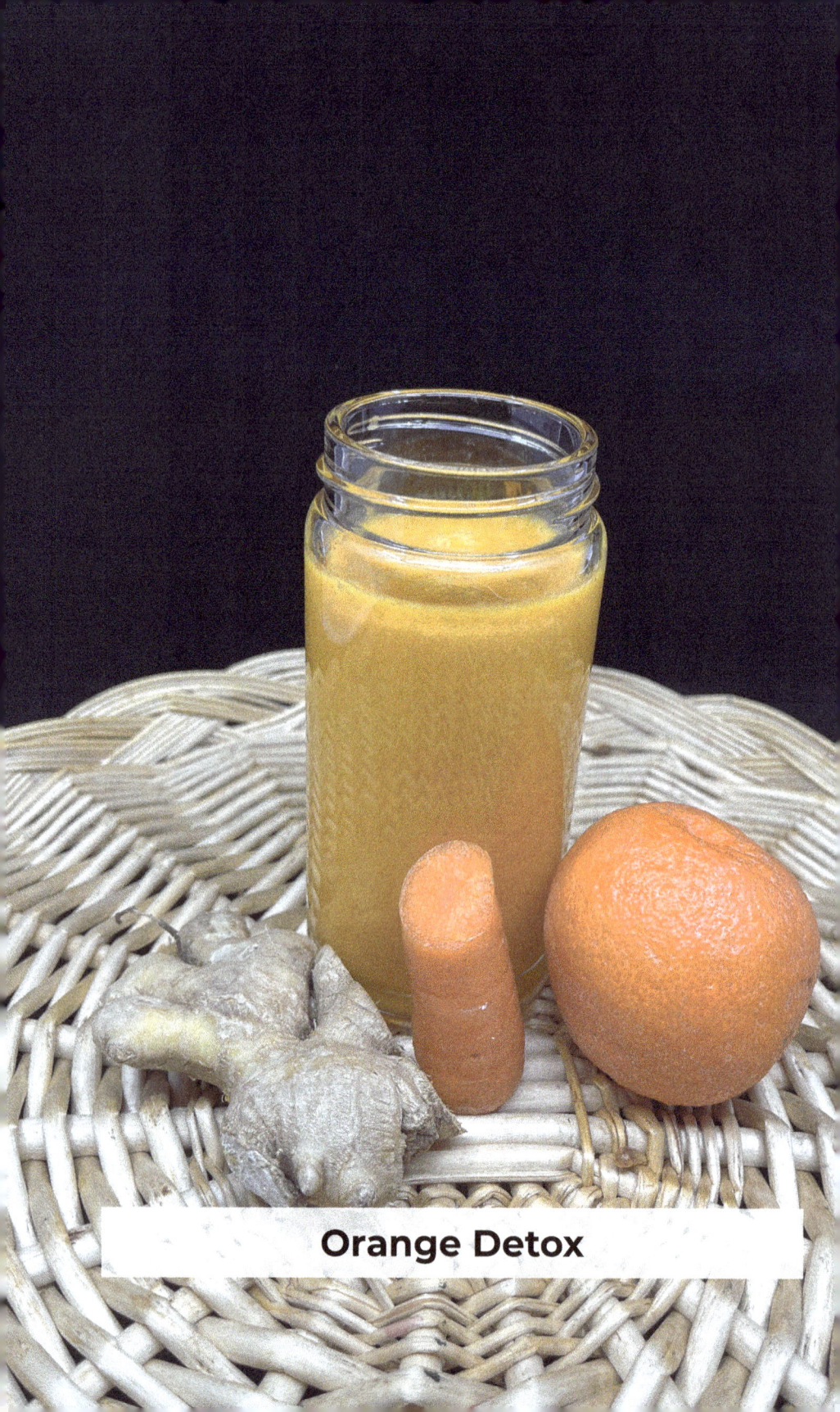
Orange Detox

DX2. Orange Detox

Ignite your senses with my zesty Orange Detox smoothie! Oranges, turmeric, and carrots lower blood pressure, reduce inflammation, and protect cells. Ginger adds a spicy twist, while flax seeds offer omega-3 and protein powder. Feel the detoxifying effects as you nourish your body and tone your muscles. Savor the revitalizing goodness in every sip!

INGREDIENTS

🛎️ (Serves 1)

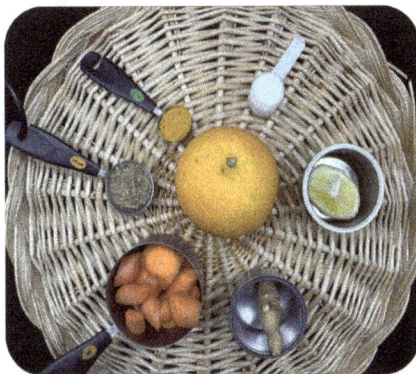

- » 1 large orange (seedless, peeled)
- » 1 cup shredded carrots
- » 2 tablespoons flax seeds grounded.
- » 3-inch piece ginger (thinly sliced)
- » 1 scoop whey protein powder (if you are not allergic to milk) or collagen powder.
- » ¼ cup lemon juice
- » ½ cup water
- » 1 teaspoon of turmeric (or 3 slides of turmeric root)

INSTRUCTIONS

1. Place all ingredients in a high-speed blender and puree until smooth. Add more ice to thicken until you've reached the desired consistency.
2. BON APPETITE!

Orange Detox's Ingredients

Orange Detox Smoothie nutrition facts and benefits

NUTRITION FACTS
(1 serving)

Calories: 271kcal
Carbohydrates: 29g
Protein: 26g
Fat: 6g
Saturated Fat: 1g
Cholesterol: 73mg
Sodium: 143mg
Potassium: 631mg
Fiber: 6g
Sugar: 14g

HEALTH BENEFITS: Ginger is packed with gingerols, paradols, sesquiterpenes, shogaols, and zingerone, all of which have powerful anti-inflammatory and antioxidant properties [6]. Hesperidin is a citrus flavonoid that is one of the key antioxidants in oranges and may lower blood pressure, reduce inflammation, and protect cells from free radical damage [132]. he benefits of Whey Protein combined with resistance training and a reduction in overall calorie consumption [133]. Collagen is the central structural component of extracellular connective tissue, which provides elastic qualities to tissues [134].

Most nutrition experts recommend ground over whole flaxseed because the ground form is easier to digest. Flaxseed is commonly used to improve digestive health or relieve constipation. Flaxseed may also help lower total blood cholesterol. Curcumin (Turmeric) has been studied extensively for its potential anti-inflammatory, antioxidant, and anti-cancer properties.

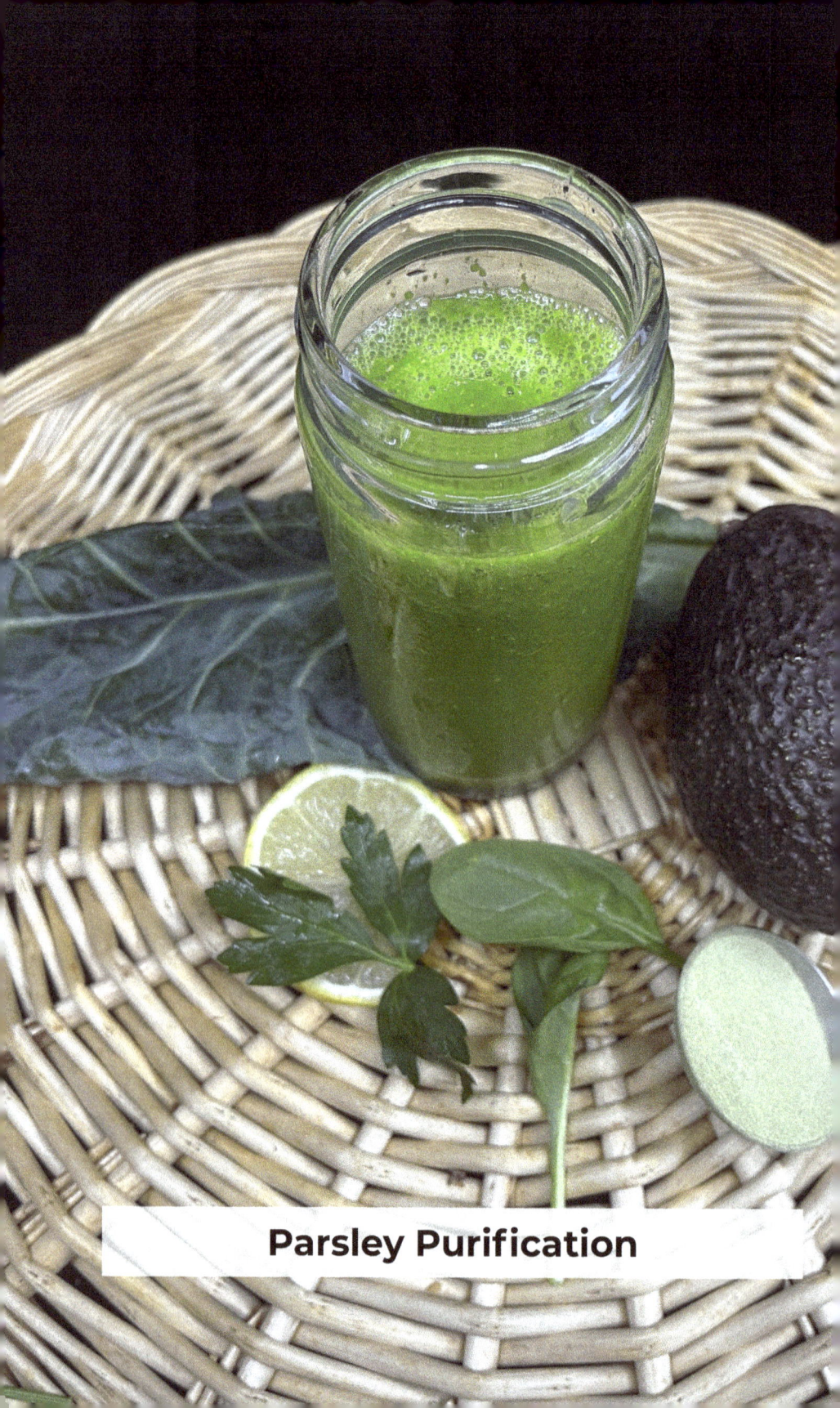
Parsley Purification

DX3. Parsley Purification

Experience the purification benefits of our Parsley Purification smoothie! Moringa's nutritional goodness protects, while avocado, pineapple, and collard greens support your healthy diet. The potent properties of parsley blend delightfully, leaving you refreshed and renewed. Matcha adds a rich flavor and regulates the microbiota. Savor the revitalizing goodness and elevate your well-being to new heights!

INGREDIENTS

🍽 (Serves 1)

» 1 cup packed raw baby spinach (approx. 1¼ oz.)
» ½ cup collar green or kale
» ¼ cup parsley shopped
» 1 scoop moringa powder
» 1 scoop of matcha powder
» 1/4 ripe avocado
» 1/2 fresh lime, juiced (approx. 2 tablespoons)
» 1/3 cup frozen pineapple
» 1½ cups water

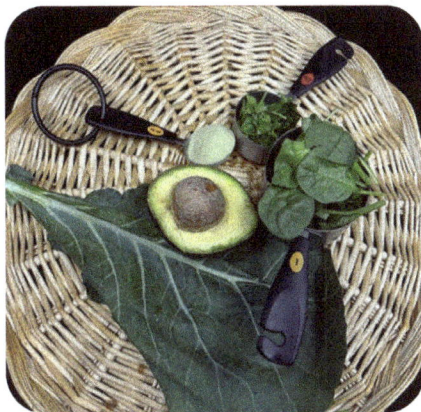

INSTRUCTIONS

1. Add all the ingredients to a blender. If the drink is too thick, add 5 ice cubes and pulse a few times.
2. Taste for sweetness and add raw honey or a date.
3. Just whisk it before drinking

Parsley Purification's Ingredients

Parsley Purification nutrition facts and benefits

NUTRITION FACTS
(1 serving)

Calories: 126kcal
Carbohydrates: 10g 1
Protein: 2.2g
Fat: 10g
Saturated Fat: 1.5g
Cholesterol: 17.5mg
Sodium: 16mg
Potassium: 313.2mg
Fiber: 5.3g
Sugar: 1.4g

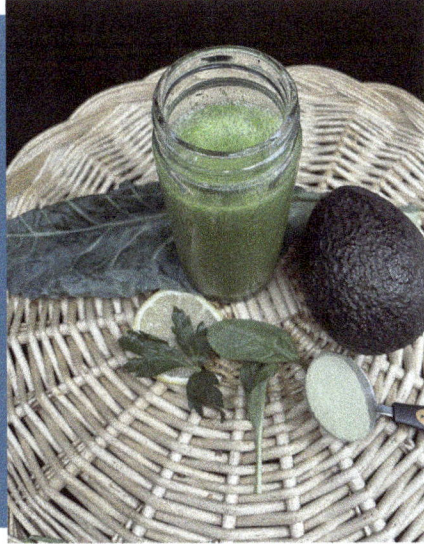

HEALTH BENEFITS: Spinach packs high amounts of antioxidants, which may also fight cancer [23]. Zeaxanthin and lutein in spinach work to prevent macular degeneration and cataracts, which are major causes of blindness [24]. Studies have shown that parsley seems to increased levels of erythrocyte glutathione reductase and superoxide dismutase. It has also been shown that parsley offers purification benefits [135]. Moringa consumption may overcome the nutritional imbalances of daily modern households, preventing the emergence of hypertension and diabetes [136]. Matcha helps to modulate the microbiota [137].

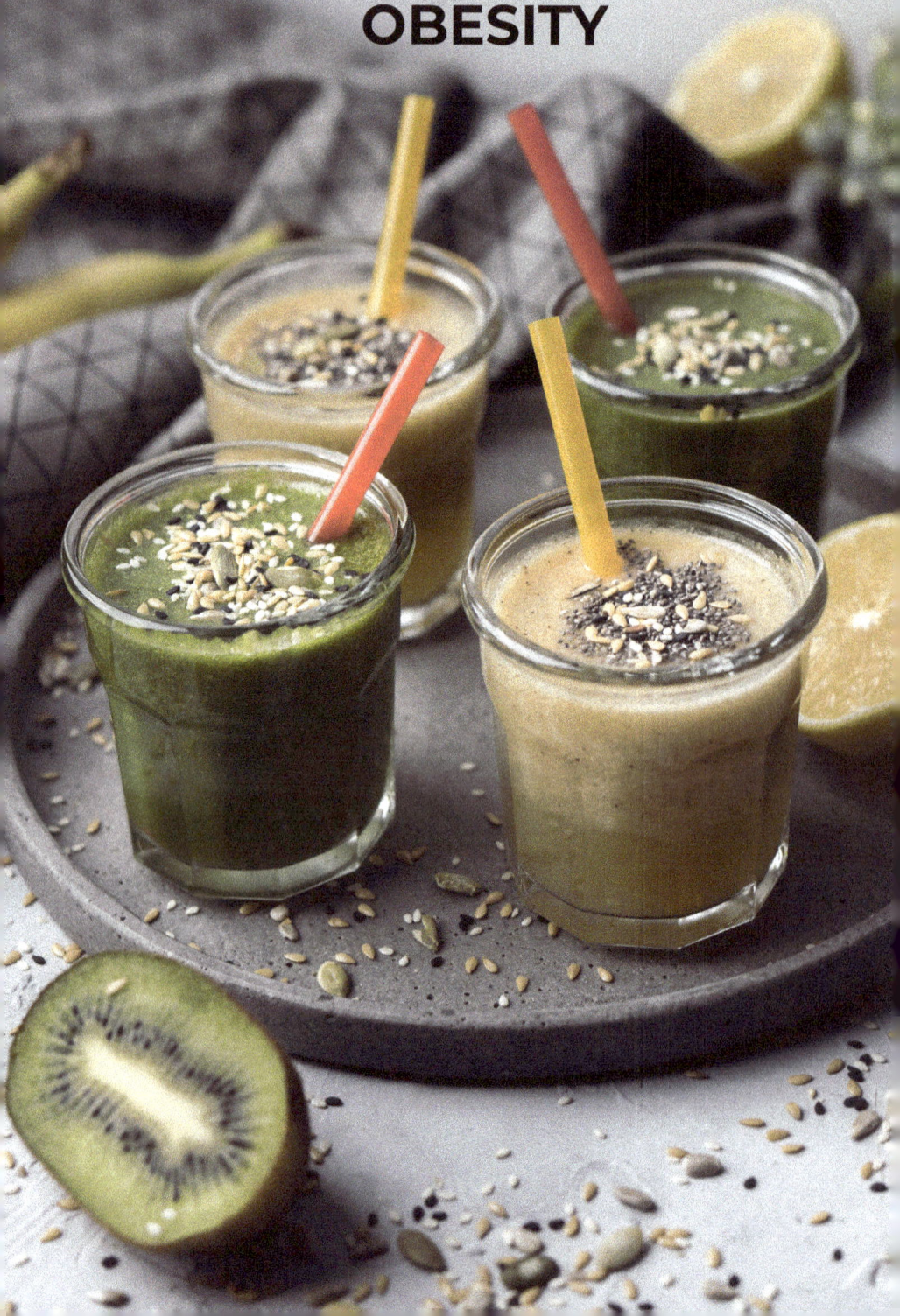

SMOOTHIES TO FIGHT OBESITY

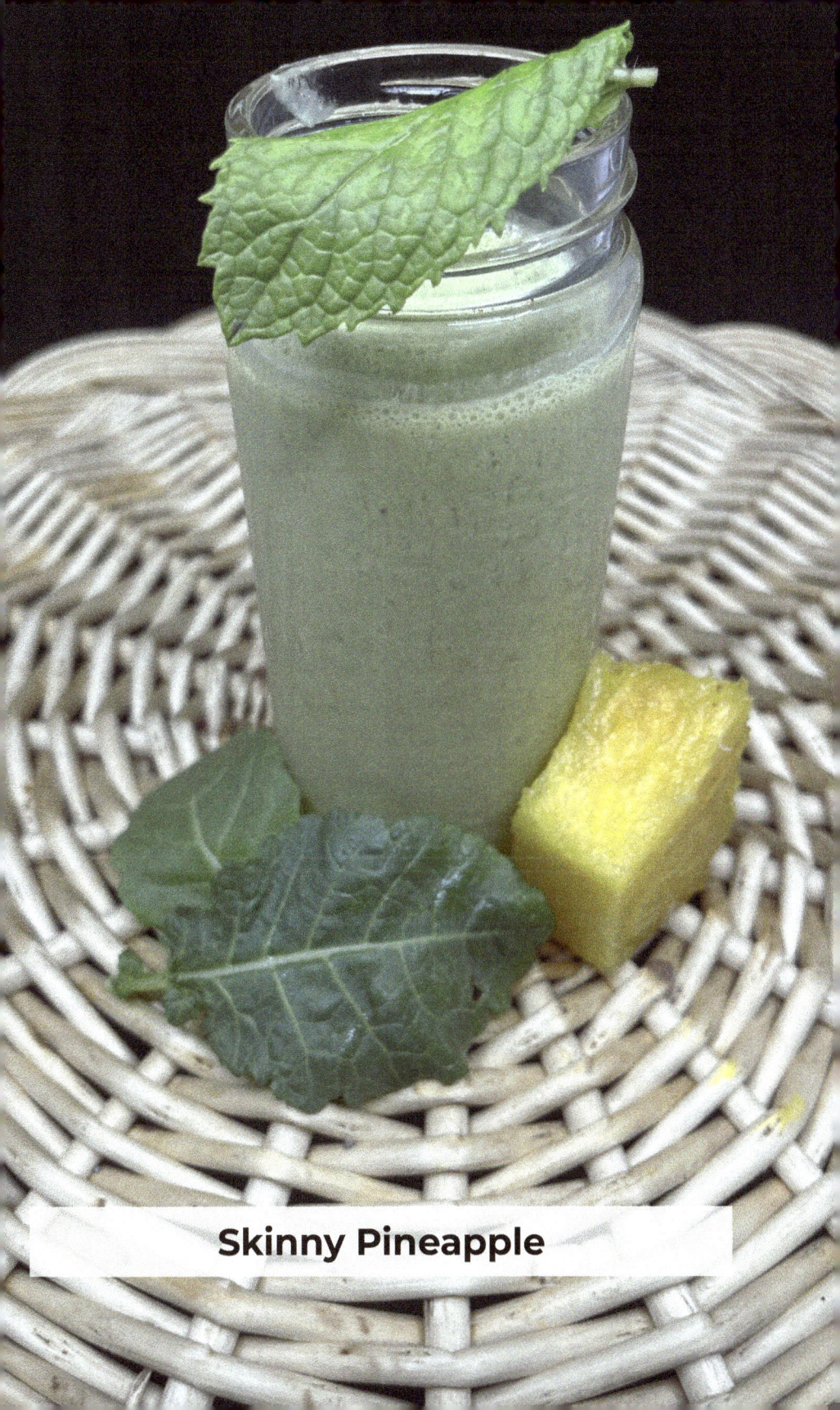

Skinny Pineapple

WM1. Skinny Pineapple

Uncover the secrets of weight management with the Skinny Pineapple smoothie! Pineapple, cultured low-fat milk probiotics, nuts, and spinach combine to protect your microbiota and support metabolic health. Enjoy the journey to a revitalized body and enhanced well-being with each sip of this nourishing blend!

INGREDIENTS

(Serves 1)

» 1 cup of pineapple chunks (you can use frozen pineapple instead)
» 1 leaf small leaf of sprig fresh mint
» ½ cup plain cultured low-fat milk probiotic (kefir) or cultured plant-based milk (contains probiotic)
» ¼ teaspoon vanilla extract
» ½ cup baby kale or baby spinach
» 1 tablespoon flax seeds grounded
» 5 half pecans or 5 half walnuts
» ¼ cup rolled oats
» ½ cup of ice cubes, add 1/3 cup of water if needed

INSTRUCTIONS

1. Add the pineapple chunks, leaf small leaf of sprig fresh mint, ½ cup kefir, ¼ teaspoon vanilla extract, baby kale, 1 tablespoon flax seed, pecans, and the rolled oats.
2. Blend until fully incorporated and creamy. You shouldn't see the texture of the solids; everything should be as smooth as possible.
3. Taste and add extra mint leaves if you want a more minty taste.
4. BON APPETITE!

Skinny Pineapple's Ingredients

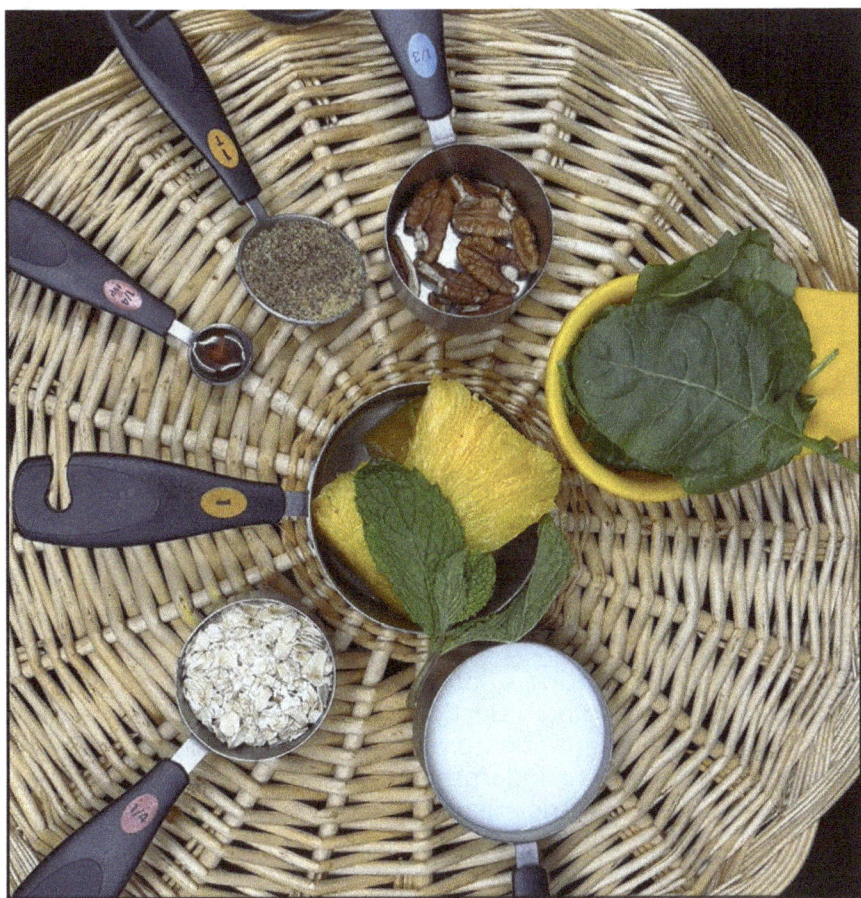

Skinny Pineapple nutrition facts and benefits

NUTRITION FACTS
(1 serving)

Calories: 438kcal
Carbohydrates: 58g
Protein: 24g
Fat: 14g
Saturated Fat: 1g
Cholesterol: 8mg
Sodium: 100mg
Potassium: 663mg
Fiber: 9g
Sugar: 29g

HEALTH BENEFITS: Pineapples contain other micronutrients, such as copper, thiamine, and vitamin B6, which are essential for healthy metabolism (important for losing that extra weight) [10]. Flaxseed is particularly high in thiamine, a B vitamin that plays a key role in energy metabolism [30]. Research is beginning to show that eating a lot of nuts leads to greater weight loss and overall lower body weights than eating a lot less nuts [34]. Vanilla extract has demonstrated anti-aging efficacy and might provide a substantial benefit in the daily care of naturally aged skin in women, through its synergistic effect on inflammation. vanilla curbs sugar intake [138]. Kefir protects gastric microbiota and metabolic health [139].

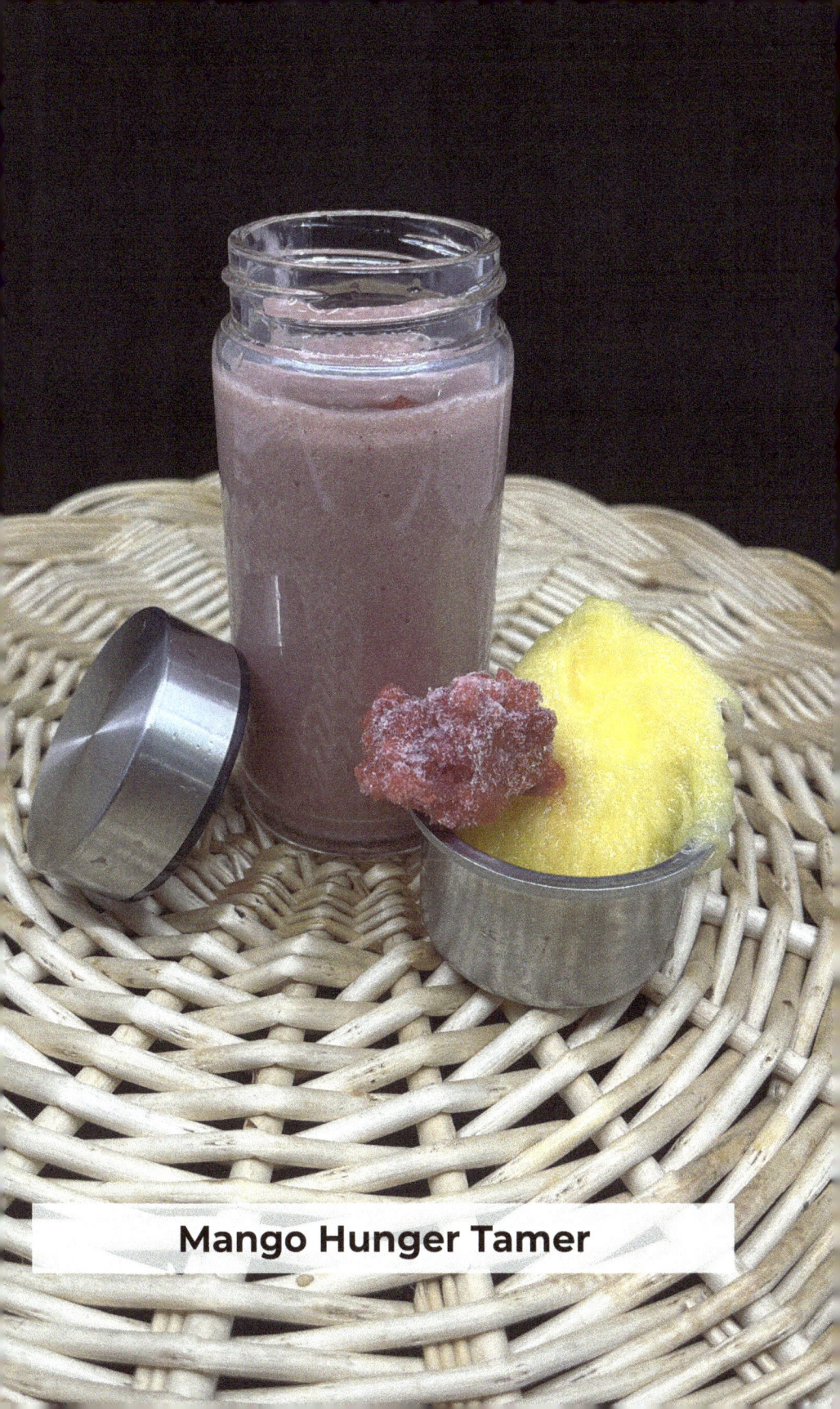

Mango Hunger Tamer

WM2. Mango Hunger Tamer

Satisfy your yearning with this tantalizing smoothie to calm down hunger! Mango and raspberries work their magic, offering nutrient-dense and fiber-rich goodness. You can then enhance it with your favorite protein, be it whey or collagen, and the calming effects of maca. Relish this fulfilling blend and experience a truly satiating delight!

INGREDIENTS

🛎 (Serves 1)

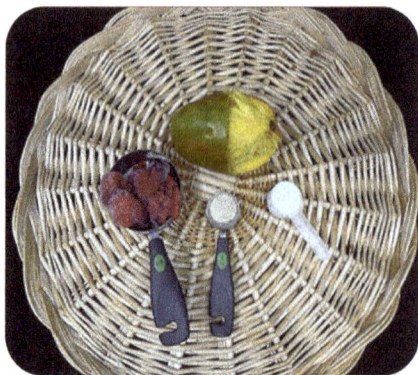

» 1/2 cup of frozen mango or 1 mango (no seed)
» ½ cup of raspberry (frozen or not)
» 1 cup almond milk or water
» 1 scoop of your favorite protein (whey or collagen)
» 1 teaspoon maca powder

INSTRUCTIONS

1. Add all ingredients in the jar and blend till you get a smooth consistency.
2. Pour in a glass and serve immediately.
3. BON APPETITE!

Mango Hunger Tamer's Ingredients

Mango Hunger Tamer nutrition facts and benefits

NUTRITION FACTS
(1 serving)

Calories: 253kcal
Carbohydrates: 28g
Protein: 28g
Fat: 6g
Saturated Fat: 1g
Cholesterol: 50mg
Sodium: 372mg
Potassium: 367mg
Fiber: 6g
Sugar: 21g

HEALTH BENEFITS: According to one study, eating fresh fruit like mango at the beginning of a meal may prevent you from overeating later on [140]. One cup (123 grams) of raspberries has only 64 calories and 8 grams of fiber. What's more, it's made up of more than 85% water. This makes raspberries a filling, low-calorie food. Compared to casein and soy proteins, whey protein seems to be more satiating. For those who need to eat fewer calories and reduce weight, these characteristics make it very helpful [141]. Research has revealed that maca is beneficial to social memory and that it restores social recognition impairments by augmenting the oxytocinergic neuronal pathways, which play an essential role in diverse social behaviors [78].

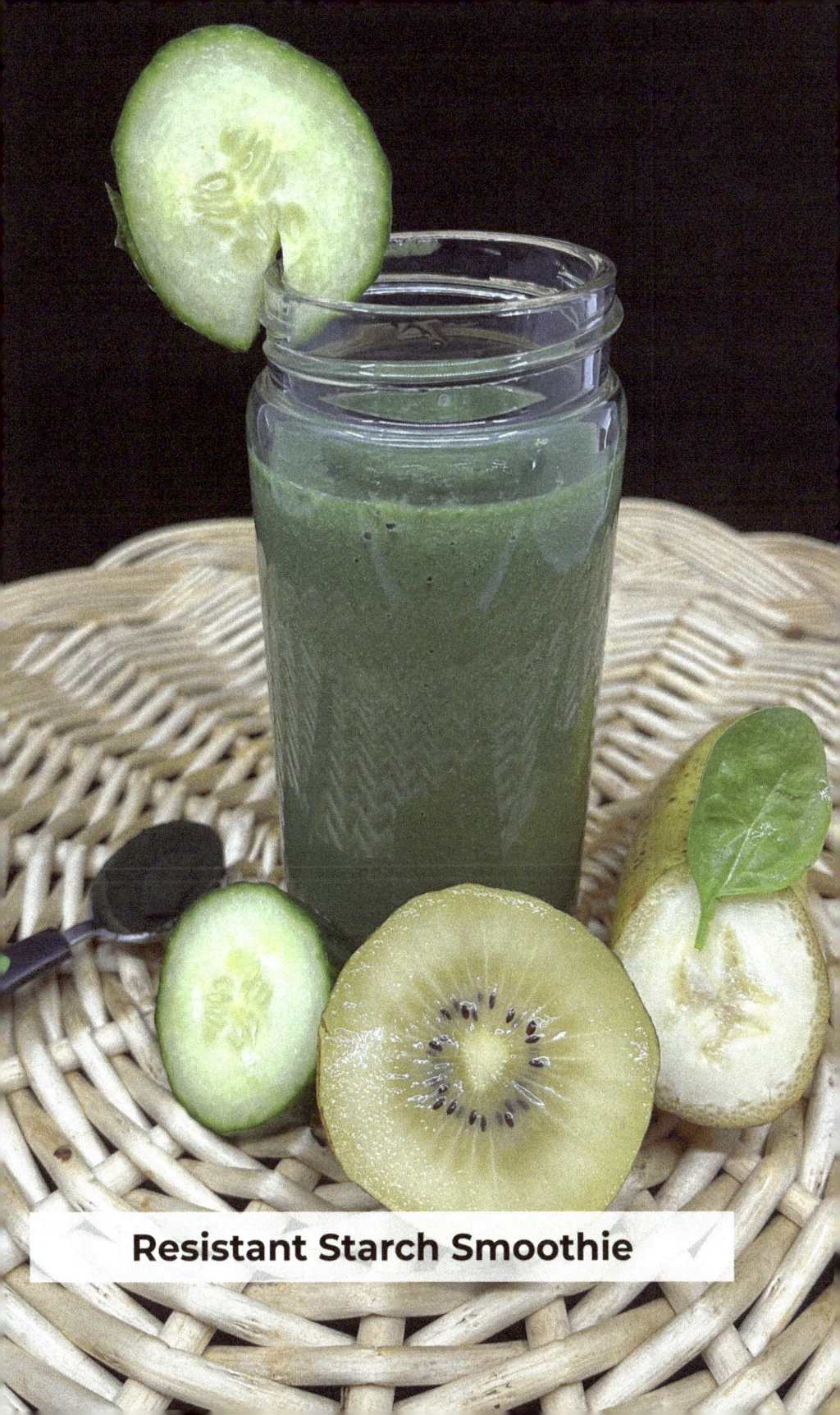
Resistant Starch Smoothie

WM3. Resistant Starch Smoothie

Unleash the power of resistant starch with the resistant Starch smoothie! Cucumbers, spinach, and fruits like pineapple, unripe banana, kiwi, and avocado offer fiber and essential nutrients for weight loss. Spirulina's protein brings a nutrient-dense boost, supplying essential amino acids. Conquer your appetite and achieve your weight loss goals with this empowering blend!

INGREDIENTS

🍽 (Serves 1)

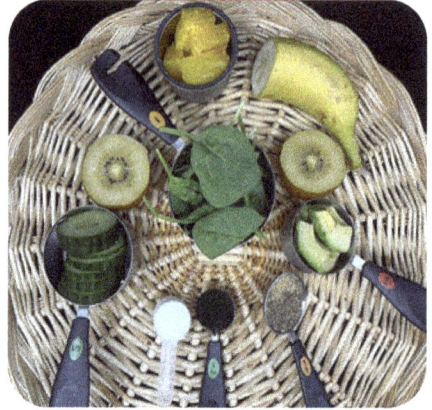

» 1 cup baby greens (spinach, kale, arugula, etc.)
» 3/4 cup frozen mango or pineapple chunks
» 1/2 unripe banana
» 1/2 cup cucumber or frozen zucchini
» 1/4 cup frozen avocado chunks
» 1 kiwi
» 1 tablespoon ground flax seed
» 1 teaspoon spirulina powder
» 1 cup unsweetened almond milk or water
» 1 scoop protein or collagen powder (optional)

INSTRUCTIONS

1. Combine all of the ingredients in a high-powered blender until smooth and creamy.
2. Pour into a glass or bowl and enjoy as it is or with your favorite smoothie bowl toppings.
3. BON APPETITE!

Resistant Starch
Smoothie's Ingredients

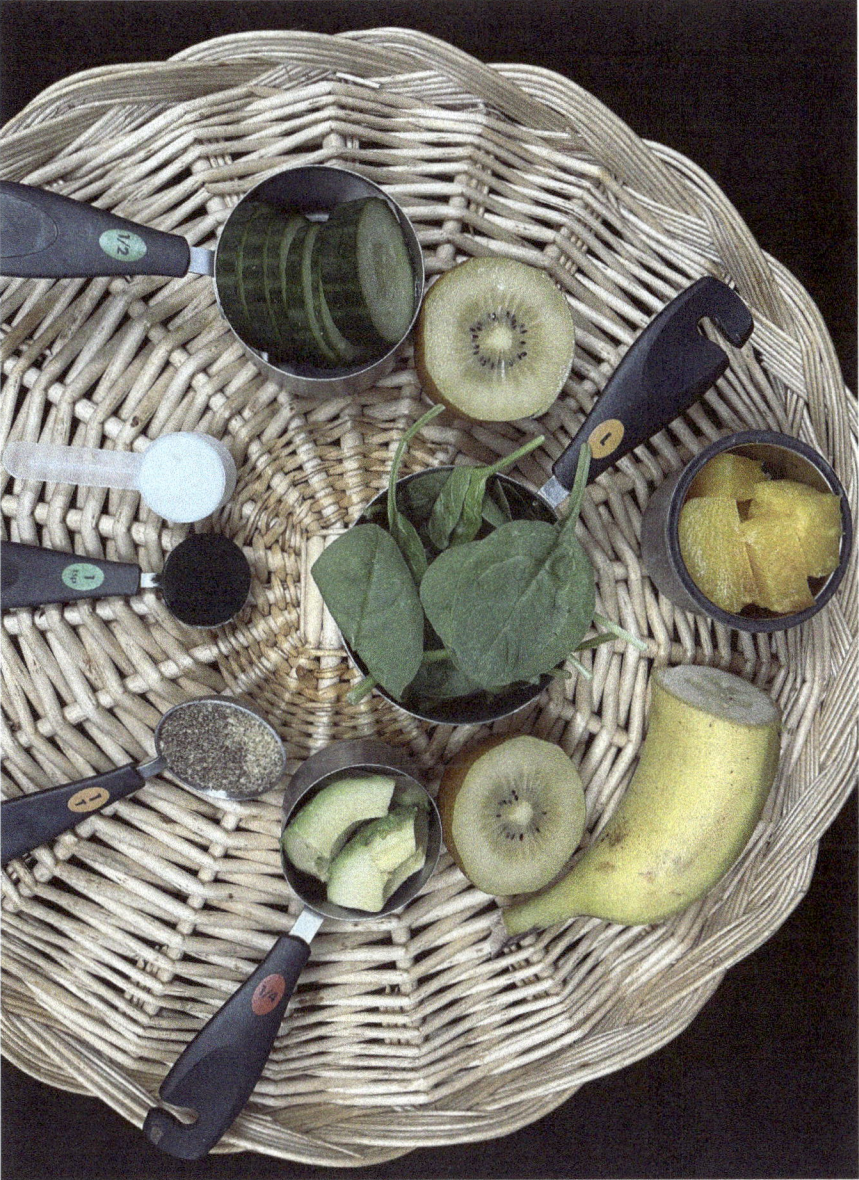

Resistant Starch Smoothie nutrition facts and benefits

**NUTRITION FACTS
(1 serving)**

Calories: 290kcal
Carbohydrates: 39g
Protein: 23g
Fat: 8g
Saturated Fat: 1g
Cholesterol: 3mg
Sodium: 63mg
Fiber: 11g
Sugar: 20g

HEALTH BENEFITS: The two types of fiber in banana may moderate your blood sugar levels after meals. Plus, they may help regulate your appetite by slowing the emptying of your stomach. More fiber from fruits and vegetables has been frequently related to reduced body weight. Unripe bananas are also loaded with resistant starch, which makes them full and helps you feel less hungry. Try preparing unripe bananas the same way you would plantains if you want to incorporate them into your diet [142] [143]. Blue-green algae, such as spirulina, may thrive in both fresh and salt water. It is a fantastic source of protein, copper, and B vitamins and is quite nutrient-dense. Moreover, spirulina's protein is of great quality and contains all the important amino acids your body requires [28].

Nourshing Reflections

Embarking on this journey of 'A Makeover to takeover your Health: Research-based Smoothies' has been an incredible experience, and we've covered three vital 'N's - Nourish your Mind, Nourish your Body, and Nourish your Soul. As we reach the end of this transformative path, it's time to bid you farewell with best wishes for your wellness journey ahead.

A word about 'Nourish your Mind,' you've laid the foundation by perceiving and preparing. You've taken the crucial steps of self-awareness, identifying strengths, areas for improvement, and crafting a wellness plan that's uniquely yours. Keep nurturing this mental resilience as you continue forward.

The book is focused on using smoothies to 'Nourish your Body', this marks your commitment to becoming the healthy individual you aspire to be. You've armed yourself with knowledge, understanding the needs and strengths of your body, and making informed choices about nutrition, exercise, and rest. Remember, you have the power to fuel your body for a healthier, happier you.

Finally, 'Nourish your Soul' is about maintaining emotional health and cultivating positive connections. You've learned to promote self-care, manage stress, and practice meditation. As you embark on this new chapter, surround yourself with supportive individuals and stay consistent in your efforts. You've got this, and your soul deserves to flourish.

As you leave the pages of this book, remember that 'A Makeover to Takeover your Health' is not just an ordinary collection of smoothie recipes. It's a result of careful curation, extensive research, and a dedication to premium ingredients. You'll find detailed insights into the benefits of each smoothie in the "health benefits" section, designed to simplify your journey to wellness.

The measurements and portions provided are typically enough for one to two servings, making it easier for you to integrate these nutritious smoothies into your daily routine.

With a heart full of hope and the belief in your ability to make positive changes, I say goodbye and wish you all the best on your path to better health. May these smoothie recipes be your allies in nourishing your soul, your body, and your mind. Farewell and good luck!"

About the Author

Dr. Elsa-Sofia Morote proudly holds two doctoral degrees and boasts a distinguished background as a senior postdoc at Massachusetts Institute of Technology. As a higher education executive, previously serving as dean in two different universities, her accomplishments are both extensive and impressive. With over 50 peer-reviewed articles, books, and book chapters, as well as mentoring 200 dissertations, she is a prolific researcher and educator, deserving of accolades.

A best-selling author, her series "A Makeover to Takeover" empowers readers to unlock their full potential and happiness. Her latest addition, "A Makeover to Takeover Your Health," stems from her personal journey of conquering autoimmune diseases and embracing healthy habits, leading to a remarkable weight loss of 30 pounds. This transformative experience served as the inspiration to share her knowledge, guiding others to nourish themselves mentally, physically, and spiritually.

Completing a health and wellness certificate at Harvard University Medical School, Dr. Morote has since embraced a life dedicated to lifestyle medicine. Alongside her role as a Professor of Public Management at John Jay College of Criminal Justice, she serves as President of the Dowling International Academy, a non-profit organization dedicated to advancing leaders and scholars, aiming for the 3 I's: Inquiry, Innovation, and Impact, to improve the well-being of society.

"A Makeover to Takeover Your Health" envisions creating nutrition awareness to improve the well-being of humanity by developing and promoting dietary guidance. Dr. Morote's work and advocacy leave a lasting, positive impact on individuals and communities alike, and she takes great pride in fostering healthier, happier lives for all.

REFERENCES

1. Cordero, D.A., Jr., *Enhancement of Virtues: Key to a Healthy Lifestyle against Chronic Diseases and Future Health Crisis.* **Korean J Fam Med, 2023.**
2. Jaqua, E., et al., *The Impact of the Six Pillars of Lifestyle Medicine on Brain Health.* Cureus, 2023. **15**(2): p. e34605.
3. Nadolsky, K., A. Baraki, and S. Nadolsky, *"Incorporating a Gym Facility in a Lifestyle Medicine Practice for Patients with Diabetes Mellitus".* Am J Lifestyle Med, 2023. **17**(3): p. 386-396.
4. Sears, B. and A.K. Saha, *Dietary Control of Inflammation and Resolution.* Frontiers in nutrition (Lausanne), 2021. **8**: p. 709435-709435.
5. Fatahi, S., et al., *The effects of almond consumption on inflammatory biomarkers in adults: A systematic review and meta-analysis of randomized clinical trials.* 2022. **13**(5): p. 1462-1475.
6. Mashhadi, N.S., et al., *Anti-oxidative and anti-inflammatory effects of ginger in health and physical activity: review of current evidence.* 2013. **4**(Suppl 1): p. S36.
7. Narai-Kanayama, A., et al., *Evidence of increases of phytol and chlorophyllide by enzymatic dephytylation of chlorophylls in smoothie made from spinach leaves.* J Food Sci, 2023. **88**(6): p. 2385-2396.
8. Sharma, G.N., G. Gupta, and P.J.C.R.i.E.G.E. Sharma, *A comprehensive review of free radicals, antioxidants, and their relationship with human ailments.* 2018. **28**(2).
9. Stewart, L.K., et al., *Quercetin transiently increases energy expenditure but persistently decreases circulating markers of inflammation in C57BL/6J mice fed a high-fat diet.* 2008. **57**: p. S39-S46.
10. Myint, Z.W., et al., *Copper deficiency anemia.* 2018. **97**: p. 1527-1534.
11. Bolling, B.W., et al., *Tree nut phytochemicals: composition, antioxidant capacity, bioactivity, impact factors. A systematic review of almonds, Brazils, cashews, hazelnuts, macadamias, pecans, pine nuts, pistachios and walnuts.* 2011. **24**(2): p. 244-275.
12. Schweiggert, R.M., et al., *Carotenoids are more bioavailable from papaya than from tomato and carrot in humans: a randomised cross-over study.* 2014. **111**(3): p. 490-498.
13. Lebaka, V.R., et al., *Nutritional composition and bioactive compounds in three different parts of mango fruit.* 2021. **18**(2): p. 741.

14. Cardoso, P.C., et al., *Vitamin C and carotenoids in organic and conventional fruits grown in Brazil.* 2011. **126**(2): p. 411-416.
15. Sierra, J.A., et al., *Consumption of golden berries (Physalis peruviana L.) might reduce biomarkers of oxidative stress and alter gut permeability in men without changing inflammation status or the gut microbiota.* Food Res Int, 2022. **162**(Pt A): p. 111949.
16. Skrovankova, S., et al., *Bioactive compounds and antioxidant activity in different types of berries.* 2015. **16**(10): p. 24673-24706.
17. He, Y., et al., *Curcumin, inflammation, and chronic diseases: how are they linked?* 2015. **20**(5): p. 9183-9213.
18. Shoba, G., et al., *Influence of piperine on the pharmacokinetics of curcumin in animals and human volunteers.* 1998. **64**(04): p. 353-356.
19. Ullah, R., et al., *Nutritional and therapeutic perspectives of Chia (Salvia hispanica L.): a review.* 2016. **53**(4): p. 1750-1758.
20. Wang, S., et al., *Biological properties of 6-gingerol: a brief review.* 2014. **9**(7): p. 1934578X1400900736.
21. Hossain, M.L., et al., *Design, Preparation, and Physicochemical Characterisation of Alginate-Based Honey-Loaded Topical Formulations.* Pharmaceutics, 2023. **15**(5).
22. Al-Kafaween, M.A., R.M. Al-Groom, and A.B.M. Hilmi, *Comparison of the antimicrobial and antivirulence activities of Sidr and Tualang honeys with Manuka honey against Staphylococcus aureus.* Iran J Microbiol, 2023. **15**(1): p. 89-101.
23. Linnewiel-Hermoni, K., et al., *The anti-cancer effects of carotenoids and other phytonutrients resides in their combined activity.* 2015. **572**: p. 28-35.
24. Vu, H.T., et al., *Lutein and zeaxanthin and the risk of cataract: the Melbourne visual impairment project.* 2006. **47**(9): p. 3783-3786.
25. Menon, V.P., et al., *Antioxidant and anti-inflammatory properties of curcumin.* 2007: p. 105-125.
26. Navaei-Alipour, N., et al., *The effects of honey on pro-and anti-inflammatory cytokines: A narrative review.* 2021. **35**(7): p. 3690-3701.
27. Ciacci, C., et al., *The kiwi fruit peptide kissper displays anti-inflammatory and anti-oxidant effects in in-vitro and ex-vivo human intestinal models.* Clin Exp Immunol, 2014. **175**(3): p. 476-84.
28. Papanikolaou, Y. and V.L. Fulgoni, 3rd, *Mango Consumption Is Associated with Improved Nutrient Intakes, Diet Quality, and Weight-Related Health Outcomes.* Nutrients, 2021. **14**(1).
29. Abuzinadah, M.F., et al., *Exploring the Binding Interaction of Active Compound of Pineapple against Foodborne Bacteria*

and Novel Coronavirus (SARS-CoV-2) Based on Molecular Docking and Simulation Studies. Nutrients, 2022. **14**(15).

30. Dzuvor, C.K.O., et al., *Bioprocessing of functional ingredients from flaxseed*. 2018. **23**(10): p. 2444.

31. Amssayef, A. and M. Eddouks, *Antihyperglycemic Effect of the Moroccan Collard Green (Brassica oleracea var. viridis) in Streptozotocin-Induced Diabetic Rats*. Endocr Metab Immune Disord Drug Targets, 2021. **21**(6): p. 1043-1052.

32. Arasu, M.V. and N.A. Al-Dhabi, *In vitro antifungal, probiotic, and antioxidant functional properties of a novel Lactobacillus paraplantarum isolated from fermented dates in Saudi Arabia*. J Sci Food Agric, 2017. **97**(15): p. 5287-5295.

33. Khanam, M., et al., *Effects of Moringa oleifera leaves on hemoglobin and serum retinol levels and underweight status among adolescent girls in rural Bangladesh*. Front Nutr, 2022. **9**: p. 959890.

34. Xu, Y., G. Chen, and M. Guo, *Potential Anti-aging Components From Moringa oleifera Leaves Explored by Affinity Ultrafiltration With Multiple Drug Targets*. Front Nutr, 2022. **9**: p. 854882.

35. Kala, K., et al., *Effect of conservation methods on the bioaccessibility of bioelements from in vitro-digested edible mushrooms*. J Sci Food Agric, 2021. **101**(8): p. 3481-3488.

36. Li, L.P., R.; Eitenmiller, R.; Chun, J.; Kerrihard, A., *Selected nutrient analyses of fresh, fresh-stored, and frozen fruits and vegetables*. Journal of Food Composition and Analysis, 2017. **59**: p. 8-17.

37. Liang, J., et al., *Influence of peeling on volatile and non-volatile compounds responsible for aroma, sensory, and nutrition in ginger (Zingiber officinale)*. Food Chem, 2023. **419**: p. 136036.

38. Park, S.J., et al., *The Effects of Curcuma longa L., Purple Sweet Potato, and Mixtures of the Two on Immunomodulation in C57BL/6J Mice Infected with LP-BM5 Murine Leukemia Retrovirus*. J Med Food, 2018. **21**(7): p. 689-700.

39. Sun, J., et al., *Impact of purple sweet potato (Ipomoea batatas L.) polysaccharides on the fecal metabolome in a murine colitis model*. RSC Adv, 2022. **12**(18): p. 11376-11390.

40. Yang, J., et al., *Anti-Inflammation and Anti-Melanogenic Effects of Maca Root Extracts Fermented Using Lactobacillus Strains*. Antioxidants (Basel), 2023. **12**(4).

41. Tang, J.S., et al., *Manuka honey-derived methylglyoxal enhances microbial sensing by mucosal-associated invariant T cells*. Food Funct, 2020. **11**(7): p. 5782-5787.

42. Tonks, A.J., et al., *A 5.8-kDa component of manuka honey stimulates immune cells via TLR4*. J Leukoc Biol, 2007. **82**(5): p. 1147-55.

43. Sarma, P.P., et al., *A pharmacological perspective of banana: implications relating to therapeutic benefits and molecular docking.* Food Funct, 2021. **12**(11): p. 4749-4767.
44. Goderska, K., K. Dombhare, and E. Radziejewska-Kubzdela, *Evaluation of probiotics in vegetable juices: tomato (Solanum lycopersicum), carrot (Daucus carota subsp. sativus) and beetroot juice (Beta vulgaris).* Arch Microbiol, 2022. **204**(6): p. 300.
45. Cho, B.O., et al., *Anti-obesity effects of enzyme-treated celery extract in mice fed with high-fat diet.* J Food Biochem, 2020. **44**(1): p. e13105.
46. Liu, Z., et al., *Sea cucumber sulfated polysaccharides and Lactobacillus gasseri synergistically ameliorate the overweight induced by altered gut microbiota in mice.* Food Funct, 2023. **14**(9): p. 4106-4116.
47. Yuan, Y., L.W. Chiu, and L. Li, *Transcriptional regulation of anthocyanin biosynthesis in red cabbage.* Planta, 2009. **230**(6): p. 1141-53.
48. Khounganian, R.M., et al., *The Antifungal Efficacy of Pure Garlic, Onion, and Lemon Extracts Against Candida albicans.* Cureus, 2023. **15**(5): p. e38637.
49. Habanova, M., et al., *Modulation of Lipid Profile and Lipoprotein Subfractions in Overweight/Obese Women at Risk of Cardiovascular Diseases through the Consumption of Apple/Berry Juice.* Antioxidants (Basel), 2022. **11**(11).
50. Wu, Z., et al., *Apple Polyphenol Extract Suppresses Clostridioides difficile Infection in a Mouse Model.* Metabolites, 2022. **12**(11).
51. Rao, S.S. and R.J.M.b.d. Najam, *Young coconut water ameliorates depression via modulation of neurotransmitters: possible mechanism of action.* 2016. **31**: p. 1165-1170.
52. Cannavale, C.N., et al., *Serum lutein is related to relational memory performance.* 2019. **11**(4): p. 768.
53. Poulose, S.M., M.G. Miller, and B.J.T.J.o.n. Shukitt-Hale, *Role of walnuts in maintaining brain health with age.* 2014. **144**(4): p. 561S-566S.
54. Azab, K.S., et al., *Withania somnifera (Ashwagandha) root extract counteract acute and chronic impact of gamma-radiation on liver and spleen of rats.* Hum Exp Toxicol, 2022. **41**: p. 9603271221106344.
55. Narra, K., S.K. Naik, and A.S. Ghatge, *A Study of Efficacy and Safety of Ashwagandha (Withania somnifera) Lotion on Facial Skin in Photoaged Healthy Adults.* Cureus, 2023. **15**(3): p. e36168.
56. Kormos, W., *On call. The coconut craze. I have seen many products promoting the health benefits of coconut oil or*

coconut water. *Is there any proof of those benefits?* Harv Mens Health Watch, 2014. **18**(11): p. 2.

57. Gu, I., et al., *Chemical Composition of Volatile Extracts from Black Raspberries, Blueberries, and Blackberries and Their Antiproliferative Effect on A549 Non-Small-Cell Lung Cancer Cells.* Life (Basel), 2022. **12**(12).

58. de Oliveira, M.R.J.N.r., *The effects of ellagic acid upon brain cells: a mechanistic view and future directions.* 2016. **41**(6): p. 1219-1228.

59. Guo, S., Y. Ge, and K.J.C.C.J. Na Jom, *A review of phytochemistry, metabolite changes, and medicinal uses of the common sunflower seed and sprouts (Helianthus annuus L.).* 2017. **11**: p. 1-10.

60. Prado, E.L. and K.G.J.N.r. Dewey, *Nutrition and brain development in early life.* 2014. **72**(4): p. 267-284.

61. Matias, A.A., et al., *Protective Effect of a (Poly)phenol-Rich Extract Derived from Sweet Cherries Culls against Oxidative Cell Damage.* Molecules, 2016. **21**(4): p. 406.

62. Kimble, R., et al., *Polyphenol-rich tart cherries (Prunus Cerasus, cv Montmorency) improve sustained attention, feelings of alertness and mental fatigue and influence the plasma metabolome in middle-aged adults: a randomised, placebo-controlled trial.* Br J Nutr, 2022. **128**(12): p. 1-12.

63. Ellatif, S.A., et al., *Immunomodulatory Efficacy-Mediated Anti-HCV and Anti-HBV Potential of Kefir Grains; Unveiling the In Vitro Antibacterial, Antifungal, and Wound Healing Activities.* Molecules, 2022. **27**(6).

64. Karaji, Z.G., et al., *Swimming exercise and clove oil can improve memory by molecular responses modification and reduce dark cells in rat model of Alzheimer's disease.* Exp Gerontol, 2023. **177**: p. 112192.

65. Alfawaz, H.A., et al., *Awareness, Knowledge and Attitude towards 'Superfood' Kale and Its Health Benefits among Arab Adults.* Nutrients, 2022. **14**(2).

66. Bonyadi, N., et al., *Effect of berry-based supplements and foods on cognitive function: A systematic review.* 2022. **12**(1): p. 3239.

67. Liu, J., et al., *Network pharmacology and mechanism studies of the protective effect of ginseng against Alzheimer's disease based on Abeta pathogenesis.* Planta Med, 2023.

68. Chou, T.W., et al., *Korean red ginseng water extract produces antidepressant-like effects through involving monoamines and brain-derived neurotrophic factor in rats.* J Ginseng Res, 2023. **47**(4): p. 552-560.

69. Swarnamali, H., et al., *Coconut oil consumption and bodyweight reduction: a systematic review and meta-analysis.* Minerva Endocrinol (Torino), 2023. **48**(1): p. 76-87.
70. Mansouri, E., et al., *Effects of virgin coconut oil consumption on serum brain-derived neurotrophic factor levels and oxidative stress biomarkers in adults with metabolic syndrome: a randomized clinical trial.* Nutr Neurosci, 2023: p. 1-12.
71. Goyal, A., et al., *A Comprehensive Review on Preclinical Evidence-based Neuroprotective Potential of Bacopa monnieri against Parkinson's Disease.* Curr Drug Targets, 2022. 23(9): p. 889-901.
72. Katayama, S., H. Ogawa, and S. Nakamura, *Apricot carotenoids possess potent anti-amyloidogenic activity in vitro.* J Agric Food Chem, 2011. **59**(23): p. 12691-6.
73. Cuadrado, A., J. Bernal, and A. Munoz, *Identification of the mammalian homolog of the splicing regulator Suppressor-of-white-apricot as a thyroid hormone regulated gene.* Brain Res Mol Brain Res, 1999. **71**(2): p. 332-40.
74. Matysek, M., et al., *Can Bioactive Compounds in Beetroot/Carrot Juice Have a Neuroprotective Effect? Morphological Studies of Neurons Immunoreactive to Calretinin of the Rat Hippocampus after Exposure to Cadmium.* Foods, 2022. **11**(18).
75. Joseph, J.A., B. Shukitt-Hale, and L.M. Willis, *Grape juice, berries, and walnuts affect brain aging and behavior.* J Nutr, 2009. **139**(9): p. 1813S-7S.
76. Fei, W., et al., *Antioxidative and Energy Metabolism-Improving Effects of Maca Polysaccharide on Cyclophosphamide-Induced Hepatotoxicity Mice via Metabolomic Analysis and Keap1-Nrf2 Pathway.* Nutrients, 2022. **14**(20).
77. Zarezadeh, M., et al., *The effect of cinnamon supplementation on glycemic control in patients with type 2 diabetes or with polycystic ovary syndrome: an umbrella meta-analysis on interventional meta-analyses.* Diabetol Metab Syndr, 2023. **15**(1): p. 127.
78. Fu, P., et al., *Oral Supplementation with Maca Improves Social Recognition Deficits in the Valproic Acid Animal Model of Autism Spectrum Disorder.* Brain Sci, 2023. **13**(2).
79. Shukitt-Hale, B., et al., *Blueberries Improve Neuroinflammation and Cognition differentially Depending on Individual Cognitive baseline Status.* J Gerontol A Biol Sci Med Sci, 2019. **74**(7): p. 977-983.
80. Delgadillo-Puga, C., et al., *Pecans and Its Polyphenols Prevent Obesity, Hepatic Steatosis and Diabetes by Reducing Dysbiosis, Inflammation, and Increasing Energy Expenditure in Mice Fed a High-Fat Diet.* Nutrients, 2023. **15**(11).
81. Jansen van Rensburg, Z., et al., *Toxic Feedback Loop Involving*

Iron, Reactive Oxygen Species, alpha-Synuclein and Neuromelanin in Parkinson's Disease and Intervention with Turmeric. Mol Neurobiol, 2021. **58**(11): p. 5920-5936.

82. Ajeigbe, K.O., et al., *Effect of coconut water and milk on heat stress-induced gastrointestinal tract dysmotility in rats: Role of oxidative stress and inflammatory response.* J Food Biochem, 2022. **46**(7): p. e14129.

83. Meyers, K.J., et al., *Antioxidant and antiproliferative activities of strawberries.* J Agric Food Chem, 2003. **51**(23): p. 6887-92.

84. Ren, M., et al., *An almond-based low carbohydrate diet improves depression and glycometabolism in patients with type 2 diabetes through modulating gut microbiota and GLP-1: a randomized controlled trial.* 2020. **12**(10): p. 3036.

85. Mishima, M.D.V., et al., *Effects of Intra-Amniotic Administration of the Hydrolyzed Protein of Chia (Salvia hispanica L.) and Lacticaseibacillus paracasei on Intestinal Functionality, Morphology, and Bacterial Populations, In Vivo (Gallus gallus).* Nutrients, 2023. **15**(8).

86. More, S. and A. Pawar, *Brain Targeted Curcumin Loaded Turmeric Oil Microemulsion Protects Against Trimethyltin Induced Neurodegeneration in Adult Zebrafish: A Pharmacokinetic and Pharmacodynamic Insight.* Pharm Res, 2023. **40**(3): p. 675-687.

87. Badeli, H., et al., *Aqueous Date Fruit Efficiency as Preventing Traumatic Brain Deterioration and Improving Pathological Parameters after Traumatic Brain Injury in Male Rats.* Cell J, 2016. **18**(3): p. 416-24.

88. Ben Necib, R., et al., *Hemp seed significantly modulates the endocannabinoidome and produces beneficial metabolic effects with improved intestinal barrier function and decreased inflammation in mice under a high-fat, high-sucrose diet as compared with linseed.* Front Immunol, 2022. **13**: p. 882455.

89. Acheson, K.J., et al., *Metabolic effects of caffeine in humans: lipid oxidation or futile cycling?* 2004. 79(1): p. 40-46.

90. Wang, X., et al., *Flavonoid intake and risk of CVD: a systematic review and meta-analysis of prospective cohort studies.* 2014. **111**(1): p. 1-11.

91. Klein, A., et al., *A randomized clinical trial in psoriasis: synchronous balneophototherapy with bathing in Dead Sea salt solution plus narrowband UVB vs. narrowband UVB alone (TOMESA-study group).* J Eur Acad Dermatol Venereol, 2011. **25**(5): p. 570-8.

92. Lee, B.H., et al., *Natural sea salt consumption confers protection against hypertension and kidney damage in Dahl salt-sensitive rats.* Food Nutr Res, 2017. **61**(1): p. 1264713.

93. Mohammed, H., *Anti-inflammatory properties of raw honey and its clinical applications in daily practice.* Qatar Med J, 2022. **2022**(2): p. 27.
94. Zielinska, M., E. Luszczki, and K. Deren, *Dietary Nutrient Deficiencies and Risk of Depression (Review Article 2018-2023).* Nutrients, 2023. **15**(11).
95. Ma, X., et al., *Lactobacillus casei and Its Supplement Alleviate Stress-Induced Depression and Anxiety in Mice by the Regulation of BDNF Expression and NF-kappaB Activation.* Nutrients, 2023. **15**(11).
96. Agarwal, S., V.L. Fulgoni, 3rd, and P.F. Jacques, *Association of 100% Fruit Juice Consumption with Cognitive Measures, Anxiety, and Depression in US Adults.* Nutrients, 2022. **14**(22).
97. Abraham, A., et al., *Vitamin E and its anticancer effects.* 2019. **59**(17): p. 2831-2838.
98. Zhang, Q., et al., *Effect of prebiotics, probiotics, synbiotics on depression: results from a meta-analysis.* BMC Psychiatry, 2023. **23**(1): p. 477.
99. Alhssan, E., S.S. Ercan, and H. Bozkurt, *Effect of Flaxseed Mucilage and Gum Arabic on Probiotic Survival and Quality of Kefir during Cold Storage.* Foods, 2023. **12**(3).
100. Yegin, Z. and M. Sudagidan, *A medical and molecular approach to kefir as a therapeutic agent of human microbiota.* Int J Vitam Nutr Res, 2022.
101. Abu-Taweel, G.M. and M.G. Al-Mutary, *Pomegranate juice moderates anxiety- and depression-like behaviors in AlCl(3)-treated male mice.* J Trace Elem Med Biol, 2021. **68**: p. 126842.
102. Li, N., et al., *Iron metabolism: An emerging therapeutic target underlying the anti-Alzheimer's disease effect of ginseng.* J Trace Elem Med Biol, 2023. **79**: p. 127252.
103. Clemens, R. and B.J. van Klinken, *The future of oats in the food and health continuum.* Br J Nutr, 2014. 112 Suppl **2**: p. S75-9.
104. Alharbi, M.H., et al., *Flavonoid-rich orange juice is associated with acute improvements in cognitive function in healthy middle-aged males.* 2016. **55**: p. 2021-2029.
105. Aune, D., et al., *Dietary intake and blood concentrations of antioxidants and the risk of cardiovascular disease, total cancer, and all-cause mortality: a systematic review and dose-response meta-analysis of prospective studies.* 2018. **108**(5): p. 1069-1091.
106. Cao, F., et al., *Extraction of polysaccharides from Maca en-hances the treatment effect of 5-FU by regulating CD4(+)T cells.* Heliyon, 2023. **9**(6): p. e16495.
107. Subash, S., et al., *Effect of dietary supplementation of dates in Alzheimer's disease APPsw/2576 transgenic mice on oxidative*

stress and antioxidant status. Nutr Neurosci, 2015. **18**(6): p. 281-8.

108. Shivanandappa, T.B., et al., *Phoenix dactylifera (Ajwa Dates) Alleviate LPS-Induced Sickness Behaviour in Rats by Attenuating Proinflammatory Cytokines and Oxidative Stress in the Brain.* Int J Mol Sci, 2023. **24**(13).

109. Sandhu, A.K., et al., *Phytochemical Composition and Health Benefits of Figs (Fresh and Dried): A Review of Literature from 2000 to 2022.* Nutrients, 2023. **15**(11).

110. Yoo, H. and H.S. Kim, *Cacao powder supplementation attenuates oxidative stress, cholinergic impairment, and apoptosis in D-galactose-induced aging rat brain.* Sci Rep, 2021. **11**(1): p. 17914.

111. Yary, T., et al., *Serum dihomo-γ-linolenic acid level is inversely associated with the risk of depression. A 21-year follow-up study in general population men.* 2017. **213**: p. 151-155.

112. Guo, X.F., et al., *Apple and pear consumption and type 2 diabetes mellitus risk: a meta-analysis of prospective cohort studies.* Food Funct, 2017. **8**(3): p. 927-934.

113. El-Elimat, T., et al., *A Prospective Non-Randomized Open-Label Comparative Study of The Effects of Matcha Tea on Overweight and Obese Individuals: A Pilot Observational Study.* Plant Foods Hum Nutr, 2022. **77**(3): p. 447-454.

114. Monobe, M., et al., *Influence of continued ingestion of matcha on emotional behaviors after social stress in mice.* Biosci Biotechnol Biochem, 2019. **83**(11): p. 2121-2127.

115. Segovia-Siapco, G., et al., *Associations between Avocado Consumption and Diet Quality, Dietary Intake, Measures of Obesity and Body Composition in Adolescents: The Teen Food and Development Study.* Nutrients, 2021. **13**(12).

116. Czarnowska-Kujawska, M., et al., *Health-Promoting Nutrients and Potential Bioaccessibility of Breads Enriched with Fresh Kale and Spinach.* Foods, 2022. **11**(21).

117. Viguiliouk, E., et al., *Effect of tree nuts on glycemic control in diabetes: a systematic review and meta-analysis of randomized controlled dietary trials.* 2014. **9**(7): p. e103376.

118. Ferreira, M.d.R., et al., *Salvia hispanica L.(chia) seed improves skeletal muscle lipotoxicity and insulin sensitivity in rats fed a sucrose-rich diet by modulating intramuscular lipid metabolism.* 2020.

119. Wahdaningsih, S., et al., *Terpenoid-lupeol of red dragon fruit (Hylocereus polyrhizus) and its immunomodulatory activity.* Pak J Pharm Sci, 2020. **33**(2): p. 505-510.

120. Naomi, R., et al., *Potential Effects of Sweet Potato (Ipomoea batatas) in Hyperglycemia and Dyslipidemia-A Systematic*

Review in Diabetic Retinopathy Context. Int J Mol Sci, 2021. **22**(19).

121. Hou, Q., et al., *The metabolic effects of oats intake in patients with type 2 diabetes: A systematic review and meta-analysis.* 2015. **7**(12): p. 10369-10387.

122. Free-Manjarrez, S., et al., *Sensory and Biological Potential of Encapsulated Common Bean Protein Hydrolysates Incorporated in a Greek-Style Yogurt Matrix.* Polymers (Basel), 2022. **14**(5).

123. Nowicka, P., A. Wojdylo, and P. Laskowski, *Inhibitory Potential against Digestive Enzymes Linked to Obesity and Type 2 Diabetes and Content of Bioactive Compounds in 20 Cultivars of the Peach Fruit Grown in Poland.* Plant Foods Hum Nutr, 2018. **73**(4): p. 314-320.

124. Hruby, A., et al., *Magnesium intake, quality of carbohydrates, and risk of type 2 diabetes: results from three US cohorts.* 2017. **40**(12): p. 1695-1702.

125. Chang, C.-S., et al., *Gamma-linolenic acid inhibits inflammatory responses by regulating NF-κB and AP-1 activation in lipopolysaccharide-induced RAW 264.7 macrophages.* 2010. **33**: p. 46-57.

126. Silva, M.L., et al., *Cinnamon as a complementary therapeutic approach for dysglycemia and dyslipidemia control in type 2 diabetes mellitus and its molecular mechanism of action: A review.* 2022. **14**(13): p. 2773.

127. Manna, K., et al., *Protective effect of coconut water concentrate and its active component shikimic acid against hydroperoxide mediated oxidative stress through suppression of NF-κB and activation of Nrf2 pathway.* 2014. **155**(1): p. 132-146.

128. Loizzo, M.R., et al., *Evaluation of chemical profile and antioxidant activity of twenty cultivars from Capsicum annuum, Capsicum baccatum, Capsicum chacoense and Capsicum chinense: A comparison between fresh and processed peppers.* 2015. **64**(2): p. 623-631.

129. Miller, G.D., et al., *Effect of Vitamin C and Protein Supplementation on Plasma Nitrate and Nitrite Response following Consumption of Beetroot Juice.* Nutrients, 2022. **14**(9).

130. Tan, M.L. and S.B.S. Hamid, *Beetroot as a Potential Functional Food for Cancer Chemoprevention, a Narrative Review.* J Cancer Prev, 2021. **26**(1): p. 1-17.

131. Wang, R., et al., *Ginger Root Extract Improves GI Health in Diabetic Rats by Improving Intestinal Integrity and Mitochondrial Function.* Nutrients, 2022. **14**(20).

132. Valls, R.M., et al., *Effects of hesperidin in orange juice on blood and pulse pressures in mildly hypertensive individuals: A*

randomized controlled trial (Citrus study). 2021. **60**: p. 1277-1288.
133. Sepandi, M., et al., *Effect of whey protein supplementation on weight and body composition indicators: A meta-analysis of randomized clinical trials.* Clin Nutr ESPEN, 2022. **50**: p. 74-83.
134. Holwerda, A.M. and L.J.C. van Loon, *The impact of collagen protein ingestion on musculoskeletal connective tissue remodeling: a narrative review.* Nutr Rev, 2022. **80**(6): p. 1497-1514.
135. Nielsen, S.E., et al., *Effect of parsley (Petroselinum crispum) intake on urinary apigenin excretion, blood antioxidant enzymes and biomarkers for oxidative stress in human subjects.* Br J Nutr, 1999. **81**(6): p. 447-55.
136. Monteiro, J., et al., *Elemental composition, total fatty acids, soluble sugar content and essential oils of flowers and leaves of Moringa oleifera cultivated in Southern Portugal.* Heliyon, 2022. **8**(12): p. e12647.
137. Ye, J.H., et al., *A comprehensive review of matcha: production, food application, potential health benefits, and gastrointestinal fate of main phenolics.* Crit Rev Food Sci Nutr, **2023**: p. 1-22.
138. Bacqueville, D., et al., *Efficacy of a Dermocosmetic Serum Combining Bakuchiol and Vanilla Tahitensis Extract to Prevent Skin Photoaging in vitro and to Improve Clinical Outcomes for Naturally Aged Skin.* Clin Cosmet Investig Dermatol, 2020. **13**: p. 359-370.
139. Kairey, L., et al., *The effects of kefir consumption on human health: a systematic review of randomized controlled trials.* Nutr Rev, 2023. **81**(3): p. 267-286.
140. Greger, M.J.A.J.o.L.M., *A whole food plant-based diet is effective for weight loss: The evidence.* 2020. **14**(5): p. 500-510.
141. Pal, S., et al., *Comparative effects of whey and casein proteins on satiety in overweight and obese individuals: a randomized controlled trial.* 2014. **68**(9): p. 980-986.
142. Lin, Y., et al., *Dietary fiber intake and its association with indicators of adiposity and serum biomarkers in European adolescents: the HELENA study.* 2015. **54**: p. 771-782.
143. Patterson, M.A., et al., *Resistant starch content in foods commonly consumed in the United States: A narrative review.* 2020. **120**(2): p. 230-244.